THE
HERBAL
HOME
REMEDY
BOOK

Simple Recipes for Tinctures, Teas, Salves, Tonics, and Syrups

JOYCE A. WARDWELL

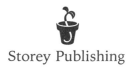
Storey Publishing

The mission of Storey Publishing is to serve our customers by publishing practical information that encourages personal independence in harmony with the environment.

Edited by Deborah Balmuth
Professional assistance from Shaitoya de la Tour
Cover and text design by Susan Bernier (based on an original design by
  Carol Jessop, Black Trout Design)
Cover illustration by Laura Tedeschi
Text production by Susan Bernier and Erin Lincourt
Drawings by Randy Mosher, Sarah Brill, and Laura Tedeschi
Indexed by Randl W. Ockey, Writeline Literary Services

© 1998 by Joyce A. Wardwell

The information in this book is true and complete to the best of our knowledge. All recommendations are made without guarantee on the part of the author or Storey Publishing. The author and publisher disclaim any liability in connection with the use of this information. For additional information please contact Storey Publishing, 210 MASS MoCA Way, North Adams, MA 01247.

Storey books are available for special premium and promotional uses and for customized editions. For further information, please call 1-800-793-9396.

Printed in the United States by Versa Press
10 9 8

Library of Congress Cataloging-in-Publication Data

Wardwell, Joyce A., 1958–
  The herbal home remedy book : simple recipes for tinctures, teas, salves, tonics, and syrups / Joyce A. Wardwell.
    p.   cm.
  Includes bibliographical references and index.
  ISBN 978-1-58017-016-1 (pbk. : alk. paper)
  1. Herbs—Therapeutic use.   I. Title.
RM666.H33W36   1998
615'.321—dc21   97-40538
                                                                   CIP

Praise for *The Herbal Home Remedy Book*

Joyce puts to print many oral traditions, which will make the learning of herbal wisdom more attractive to the young among us. A firm believer in Amerindian medicines, I'm pleased to read Joyce's recounting of some Amerindian stories, blending them skillfully with her own herbal knowledge. And it is the young among us who will carry on the herbal traditions if they learn them well. Good reading on herbal wisdom, with interesting stories that can catch the child's attention! The younger the children learn about the beauty, ease and efficacy of herbal medicine, the longer herbal medicine will survive, perhaps even overcome. I want a copy for each of my grandchildren.

— James A. (Jim) Duke,
author of *Green Pharmacy*,
Rodale Press

Just as every leaf is important to the web of wise woman, pick this leaf — this book. It is green. It is healing. It will tell you stories that weave you gently and skillfully into the ways of herbal wisdom.

— Susun Weed, author and
founder of Wise Woman Center

The story of healing with plants is a precious heritage that is made richer by The Herbal Home Remedy Book. *A spirit of connection to the earth combines in these pages with beauty and practical advice that anyone can use.*

— Amanda McQuade Crawford, MNIMH;
Dean, National College of Phytotherapy;
author of *Herbal Remedies for Women*
and *The Herbal Menopause Book*

If you're just beginning with herbs, The Herbal Home Remedy Book *is for you. This book grounds you in the fundamentals of relationship building with plants and then clearly teaches you what to do with the new plant friends you make. The abundance of Native American teaching stories adds to the joy of reading this book.*

— Pam Montgomery,
herbalist and owner of Green Terrestrial
Herbal Products, organizer of the Green
Nations Gathering, and author of
Partner Earth: A Spiritual Ecology

This book meets all my criteria for a great herb book. Written by a long-time practicing herbalist, The Herbal Home Remedy Book *explains step by patient step the skills necessary to be a self-reliant herbalist. Accentuated by the earthly wisdom of Native American stories,* The Herbal Home Remedy Book *is filled with practical herbal advice, wonderful recipes, and herbal formulas. The author suggests this is a book for beginners; I found the wisdom herein to be of value even to the more skilled herbal practitioner.*

— Rosemary Gladstar, author of
Herbal Healing for Women

Joyce Wardwell's book is a delight! The mix of herbal wisdom and storytelling is beautifully instructive and entertaining at the same time. This is a good beginner's book to overcome the feeling of being overwhelmed by herbal healing.

— Rosita Arvigo, Director of Rainforest
Remedies in Belize, Central America

DEDICATION

In memory of my great-great-grandmother Jane Wardwell, who learned her herbal craft from the Ojibway on the Minnesota frontier; and her mother, Sarah Wardwell, condemned for witchcraft in Salem, Massachusetts, on September 1, 1692; and Sarah's husband, Samuel, who was hung for witchcraft on September 22, 1692.

TABLE OF CONTENTS

ACKNOWLEDGMENTS

I'm honored to be given the opportunity to thank those who have most helped me to bring this book to you.

My editor, Deborah Balmuth, for her gentle humor, unflagging support, and skill in bringing out the best. And the publishing team at Storey for giving form to the word.

My husband and children, for aiding and abetting a crazed author.

Betsy McKenney, who kept a kind watchful eye on said children, giving me time to write.

My sisters: Dr. Marsha Pierdinock, who twenty-five years ago gave me my first guide — to wild edibles. Novice that I was, it took me two months to match a real plant to a picture, but you can't let a sister down, so I kept trying. (Now I wonder, did she do that on purpose?) And Lynette Hallmark, who enjoys digging up family roots as much as I enjoy digging up the other kind of wild roots.

Tom Brown Jr., who opened my eyes to the wonder of the wilderness.

Fellow herbalist Christa-Maria, whom I'm honored to call friend and cohort.

Barb Pratt, whose storytelling, wit, and wisdom leave an indelible imprint on all who listen.

The keepers of the Three Fires, past and present.

The countless herbalists who have walked before me and kept the traditions alive, even in the face of adversity.

And, most of all, to my mother and father, for seeing the flower in the weed.

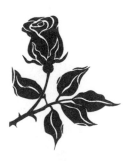

INTRODUCTION

My great-grandmother Na never went to a doctor in her life. She dismissed the doctors as charlatans, saw their medicines as harmful, and thought hospitals were places you went to die. Her back-then attitudes weren't that much different from our attitudes today, only now we mistrust shifty HMOs, spiraling hospital bills, and the side effects of drugs. Just like my grandmother, we believe that "I can do it better." One of the most famous doctors of this century, Dr. Albert Schweitzer, expressed exactly this sentiment: "It's supposed to be a professional secret, but I'll tell you anyway. We doctors do nothing. We only help and encourage the doctor within."

Indeed, roughly 80 percent of the world's population uses traditional medicine for primary health care. And lest you doubt the effectiveness of plant remedies, realize that about 30 percent of prescription drugs are still synthesized from plants. In fact, the word *drug* comes from an old Dutch word, *drogge,* which means "to dry" — a reference to the preparation of medicinal plants, of course.

Na never went to a doctor, because she had her stock of home herbal remedies. She raised three healthy children plying her craft. But her fear and mistrust of doctors also had its downside. She spent the last thirty years of her life blind with cataracts and having to sit most of the time because she had a prolapsed uterus — two conditions that modern medicine could have easily remedied. Today, we are fortunate enough to have access to the best of both worlds: We can use traditional medicine and techniques to keep ourselves healthy and prevent ailments from becoming deadly; and we can turn to either modern or alternative medicine for treatment when the crisis is beyond our capability, skills, or equipment.

CAUTION

Like any medicine, it is important to use herbs with care. The simple herbal recipes in this book are meant to inspire, and are not given as medical advice. For your individual health concerns, for chronic warning symptoms, in emergency situations, or when in doubt, seek the advice of your primary personal health care practitioner.

Twenty years ago, when I set out to learn about plants, teachers and practitioners of herbal medicine were few and far between in the United States. Happily, I was able to meet up with healers from different traditions who each dropped a clue, gave a hint, or told a story to help me on my path. But always I found myself returning to the plants themselves as my teachers. Books and teachers tell you about the plants, but the better way to learn is to work with the plants, letting them tell you about themselves.

Looking back, the path I was left to take was a fortunate gift. I was forced to develop my own way of relating to herbs and medicine. I had to seek it myself.

This book is not meant to be a complete course in herbal medicine. It is, rather, a guide to help you walk your own medicine path. Inside you'll find suggestions, options, and exercises. There is no one best way to use herbs. But if you try the various techniques within, perhaps you'll discover the one best way that works for you.

The medicine stories I share throughout this book have been guideposts in my own lifelong pursuit of herbal learning. When I became stumped or puzzled, I returned to their teachings to find a balanced perspective. Sometimes it meant unlearning all the technical information I had spent so much time accumulating. The stories remind us that there is more than one way of looking at the universe.

These stories are legends — that is, they are common to many peoples. I have heard them told and retold over campfires, in books, and in groups where each of us "knew" the true version of the tale. That is the way of a legend: It takes on a life of its own, and the life of the teller.

Sometimes, a story is so universal that it is impossible to trace it back to one original source. So I've given credit to the person, peoples, or book from which I first heard the story. These stories were a gift to me, and I am honored to have the opportunity to give them to you. They are meant to be told. It is my hope that perhaps you too will join in the cycle and pass on the gift and medicine of these stories.

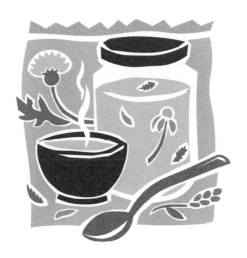

The Heart of
Herbalism:
Knowing the
Herbs

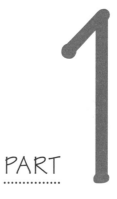

PART

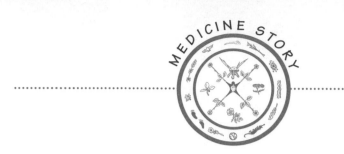

THE VIOLET GARDEN

There once was a young girl who loved violets so dearly that she'd walk miles to pick a bouquet. Her grandmother, ever practical, suggested that the young girl plant some violets nearby — it would be a good start toward a first garden. The young girl agreed, and she determined to hunt until she found the perfect violet plants.

She went to the maple forests where the violets grew wild. She went to the sunny edges where the violets grew taller. She went to the wet spots where the violets were lush and full. She hunted for the densest stand of violets she had ever found. She searched and searched until she found the perfect violet for her garden.

Right away she took her digger and began to cut the violet's roots loose. Excited, she quickly dug and pulled up on the plant to help it get free. Suddenly, the whole plant came out of the ground, and the roots were left behind! Arrghh! Now her violets would die — and her garden, too — because of a bit of carelessness. Not knowing what else to do, she bundled up the broken plant and returned to ask her grandmother for help.

"Look, Gumma, I ruined the violets for my garden!" She wailed. "I can't do anything right! How can I fix this? I don't know what to do! How can it live with no roots? How can I plant it? How much sun does it need? And what about water? What do I do?"

Gumma looked at the child squarely. She said, "It doesn't matter where you plant the violets, or how. All you need to do is to Simply Care for the plant. Pay attention, watch, and listen. Be patient. Remember to Simply Care — and all the rest you need to know will follow."

This version of the story was first told to me by my Gumma, Claire Sulem. Her father told her a slightly different version when she was learning to grow carrots for market.

CHAPTER 1
Getting to Know the Plants

Involvement is the key to understanding.
— Rolling Thunder

Herbal healing begins long before we drink a medicinal tea. It begins before we even pick the tea. Herbal healing begins when we decide to gather our own medicine. This decision empowers us and initiates the healing process. Once we step out into the fresh air, all our senses open, and we can find our plant. It is a hunt. To be successful, nature demands we listen to her and disregard our woes. We must follow clues, track ecosystems, venture into new places, breathe deep, and ease our spirits.

Herbal gathering provides an intimate connection with natural cycles that can never come from merely buying an herb. And by following a few simple guidelines, the quality of the herbs you gather will far exceed that of what you can buy, much the way an imported tomato from the local supermarket pales in comparison to the fresh-picked garden-grown kind.

LEARNING TO RECOGNIZE PLANTS

Remember a TV game show called *Name That Tune?* "I can name that tune in four notes, Dave!" But could you? And get it exactly right? Not often. And ultimately no one — not the contestants, the emcee, or the viewers — ever got to experience the whole song — just enough notes to drive them crazy.

Many of us approach field identification in the same way, only we play Name That Plant. We tote our field guides everywhere and attempt to correctly identify as many plants as possible. But it doesn't work! So we look for a teacher to take us on guided walks to help us identify as many plants as possible. Guess what? That doesn't work either. So what does?

Let me tell you a story. One summer there were so many yellow jacket nests near our home it seemed that someone was getting stung nearly every day. My six-year-old daughter, Emily, took her "job" of picking a plantain remedy quite seriously. She never let anyone else chew or even bruise the leaf before she placed it on the sting. She especially enjoyed putting the mash on her twin baby brothers' stings, because the two boys would always smile at her through their tears.

One day, when the one-year-old twins were playing, one of them got stung again, but Emily was nowhere about. So the other twin went over to the plantain patch, picked a leaf, chewed it, and placed it on the sting until the crying stopped. He didn't know the plant's name — couldn't even have said it if he had. But he didn't need a name; he knew what to look for.

To learn a plant, you must first learn to recognize it. Don't worry about its name. Call it the "Plant I Stepped on Last Tuesday" or the "Plant That Looks like My Cousin Fred" (just don't let Cousin Fred know). The purpose of a name is only to communicate to another person what plant you are talking about or to help you remember the plant. It will not teach you anything about the plant. For that, you must teach yourself!

A Beginning Exercise

Start by taking this book and a blank notebook outside with you. Find a plant you are curious about. Look at it carefully. Now draw the plant. Don't think about your third-grade art teacher; you're not being graded. But notice how the way that you look at the plant changes when you draw it. You examine it more closely, you notice spatial relationships and how light and shadow play on the leaves. This is the right side of your brain taking charge, the side in charge of creativity, instinct, and intuitive memory.

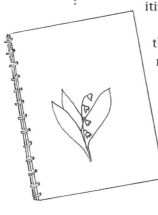

Next, hunt for another plant of the same kind as the one you just drew. Draw that one also. The plants may be of the same species, but they have individual differences that will become clearer to you as you draw.

Come back periodically to these same plants to observe how they change through the growing season. Notice how the seeds form, who pollinates the plant, what bugs or animals live on or eat the plant, how the plant looks at dusk, at dawn, after a rain, during drought. Watch.

Meanwhile, look for more of this same plant during your travels. Notice if it grows differently in sunny open places than when in the shade. Where do you usually see the plant? Perhaps you'll start to recognize other plants growing nearby. Draw them, too. Write down your homemade names under your pictures.

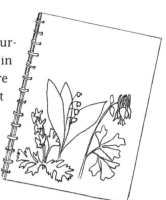

Getting Fully Acquainted

Now take a look at the plant from new and different perspectives. Imagine an ant's view of the plant; or, if it's a tree, try to climb it and see how it looks from above. Allow yourself the freedom to explore the plant and get to know it in unusual (and even impractical) ways. Pretend you are the plant by sitting upright and not moving, write a poem or a song for the plant to leave it as a gift, or make a craft from the plant.

Acquaint yourself with this one plant — just the same as you would acquaint yourself with a friend. How many people do you know when you see them, but don't remember their name? How many times do you meet them before their name sinks in? This is how many times you should acquaint yourself with a plant before you give a name to it.

WAYS OF CLASSIFYING PLANTS

Modern botanical classification groups plants by sexual (reproductive) characteristics, but there are other ways to group plants.

Native American tribes classify plants by the directions of north, south, east, and west. The Cherokee further classify plants by their function — thus there are warrior plants such as brambles and poison ivy, and scout plants such as poplar and plantain. The Anishinaabe of the Great Lakes classify by family roles: Grandmother Cedar, Grandfather Birch, and Elder Sister Balsam Fir.

The Chinese divide plants into yin and yang (female and male) as well as by taste and by the elements of wood, fire, earth, water, and metal. It is just as fascinating to explore these ways of relating to plants as it is to explore your own.

READY FOR PLANT IDENTIFICATION

Once you can recognize the plant in various settings, in various stages of growth, and at various times of day, then you are ready to take out a field guide and try to find its given name. You'll be surprised at how easy it is and how well you remember. You may have guessed the name already! Take it slow — don't try to name every plant you've been drawing on the same day.

Use a field guide that has black and white drawings. Drawings highlight specific key details in a way that no photograph can. In fact, field guides that use color photographs are often the hardest to identify from. Once you identify a plant, color it in (colored pencils work best) so you can quickly reference it again. I recommend using two different field guides as cross-references at first. Even the best of drawings can leave some niggling doubt about an identity. Be sure to always double- or even triple-check a new plant before putting it in your mouth!

A good field guide for beginners is the Peterson series. In these, plants are grouped first by flower color, then by petal shape. You start out doing a lot of page flipping, but you'll remember much information on a subconscious level. Then one day when you're walking through a field, you'll say, "Hey, wait — isn't that the viper's bugloss that was on the same page as the violets?" It's a small triumph, but a memorable one.

As you become more familiar with the plants, you start to group them by family. Now try using a field guide with a key to identify plants. Newcomb's Field Guide Series is used by many amateur botanists. It is less complex than a botany book and quicker to access than most flower-grouped field guide series.

WHAT YOU DON'T KNOW CAN KILL YOU

It is wise to learn the characteristics of the poisonous plants in your area. Some plants are extremely toxic. For example, water hemlock and pokeweed berries are poisonous even in small amounts. However, they are also relatively easy to identify and avoid if you know what to look for. Get to know the identifying traits of both safe and dangerous plants. A good field guide will show deadly plants alongside any look-alike but safe counterparts. Always take the time for positive plant identification, especially when gathering a plant that resembles a poisonous one.

GATHERING MEDICINAL PLANTS

When we gather, we become caretakers of a tremendous wild garden. Unfortunately, with the recent upsurge of interest in herbs, plant populations are being destroyed. Goldenseal and ginseng hardly exist in the wild. Echinacea, sweet grass, and wild ginger are just a few of many threatened herbs. Even common herbs are in trouble. In New York State, good stands of wild carrot are becoming hard to find. In northern Michigan, common milkweed was nearly eradicated to make life jackets during World War II. Always gather in a way that allows future growth, and gather from cultivated sources first whenever possible.

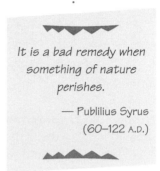

It is a bad remedy when something of nature perishes.

— Publilius Syrus (60–122 A.D.)

Protecting Future Growth

There are a few practices you can follow that will help protect plants from becoming endangered and ensure the growth of future generations. These include:

◆ Know the plant's reproductive habits before you gather. For example, a plant that reproduces from underground rhizomes should be thinned when gathering, but a plant that reproduces from seeds should be gathered sporadically, with randomly placed flowers left to turn to seed.

◆ Know what you will be using the plant for before you gather it.

◆ Gather only as much as you need.

◆ Do not wild-gather for commercial purposes.

◆ When possible, gather leaves, seeds, and flowers, which nature replaces easily, rather than barks and roots, whose loss may kill the whole plant.

◆ Do not gather endangered plants; find a substitute. For example, garlic can be used in place of goldenseal or wild echinacea for treating colds and viruses.

◆ Do not gather from wet ground. The footprints you leave compress the soil, making future growth difficult. Wait for a dry spell before gathering wetland plants.

- Leave enough for animal populations.
- Not everyone gathers with respect. Be discreet about whom you reveal your gathering spots to.
- Do not gather from sprayed areas (including marshes sprayed for mosquito control and forests sprayed for gypsy moth control), alongside roads, near factories or farms (unless it is an organic farm), or near polluted waters.

Guidelines for Gathering

Have you ever spent a day strawberry picking? Remember how the fruits were cool and chilly in the morning, but grew sweeter and juicier as the sunshine warmed them? It's important to pay attention to how the day and season affect the plant you are gathering.

Basically, you want to gather plants when they are at their peak of potency, or fully ripe. Think of the time when the plant is putting most of its energy into growing one particular part. This is the time to gather that part. Here are some useful general rules:

- **Leaves** should be gathered when they are tender and showing new growth, either before the flower buds appear, or after seeding, when new fall growth appears.
- **Flowers** are usually best before full bloom, in the mid- to late morning after the dew has dried.
- **Seeds** should be gathered when ripe and dry, but before they fall to the ground.

THE CUSTOM OF OFFERING

To place the self in a respectful attitude toward the plants and the earth, people of most cultures give a simple offering before gathering: a pinch of pollen or tobacco, a bit of water, a short song, a moment's contemplation. This small act helps us focus on the reason the plant is being gathered, ponder the cycle of life, and acknowledge our own wild essence.

- **Roots** are gathered in the early spring or late fall. Since sap rises and falls with the sun, an ideal time to gather is in the early morning or late afternoon.
- **Inner barks and saps** are best gathered in the spring when the sap is flowing, before the leaf is full size. The inner bark is gathered from the limbs of the tree, ***not*** the trunk (which can kill the tree). Midafternoon of a warm sunny day on the south-facing side of the tree is best . . . ask any maple syruper!
- **Shoots** can be gathered year-round, though spring is the preferred and most abundant time. Gather from stands that benefit from thinning.
- **Plants gathered in the spring and late fall** generally reach peak potency during cool-weather spells: Violet, rose hips, dandelion root, sun tuber, and cattail shoots are some examples.
- **Plants gathered during summer and early fall** usually need heat to develop fully and create essential oils. Gather these plants during hot spells: wild carrot seed, St.-John's-wort flower, chokecherry, sage leaf, and mullein flower.
- **Try not to gather for a day or two** after heavy rainfalls. Plants will soak up the excess moisture and lose potency.
- **Likewise, try not to gather during a drought,** as the plant cells are stressed and, again, not as potent.

If we lived in an ideal world, it would be easy to follow these guidelines 100 percent of the time. But we don't. Just because you can't gather rose hips at 3:00 in the afternoon after a hard frost on a bright sunny day three days after a rainfall doesn't mean you shouldn't gather them at all. For home medicinal purposes, cut yourself some slack.

To use as a simple tea, I have gathered poplar bark in the dead of winter and dandelion root in midsummer. Certainly their quality was not the best, but what was lacking in potency was compensated for by freshness. Perhaps I needed to use a little more of the herb — to take two cups of poplar tea instead of one. Allow yourself the freedom to explore simple and safe plants during different times of their growth. It is the only way

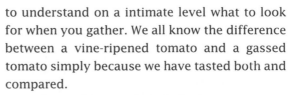
to understand on a intimate level what to look for when you gather. We all know the difference between a vine-ripened tomato and a gassed tomato simply because we have tasted both and compared.

When making medicinals for long-term storage, such as tinctures, oils, and salves, always use the best-possible-quality herb that you can gather, and make small batches until you get the feel of the medicine. There is nothing worse than having a five-year supply of ineffective tincture. It wastes your time, the plant's energy, and the money you invested, and it can even be harmful if you are relying on the tincture for medicinal purposes.

STORING HERBS

Plan to prepare your herbs for storage immediately after gathering. Herbs left to sit even overnight will degrade in quality. Shake the dirt off. Sort out dead leaves and debris. Separate stems from leaves and seeds from chaff. Wash and blot-dry roots, then spread them out to dry. Roots will need to be chopped into pieces about 1 inch thick; leaves and flowers are best left as whole as possible. There are many ways to preserve your harvest; drying, freezing, extracting, distilling, and making into a wine are just a few of the options you may wish to pursue.

Drying

Drying herbs is the easiest and most efficient way to store your harvest. It requires no special materials or equipment. All you need is a well-ventilated space out of direct sunlight and wind. The easiest way is to gather the herbs into 1-inch-diameter bundles secured with rubber bands or string to allow the air to flow through the drying plants. Then hang them in a place that is shady and dry, with good ventilation. Hanging them upside down brings the essential oils into the leaves.

Another method is to put small amounts of herbs inside paper bags. The bags absorb a fair amount of moisture and protect the herbs from sun. Shake or stir the herbs every day until dry. This is especially effective when you are drying seeds. If the plant has a lot of moisture, cut a ventilation hole at the top

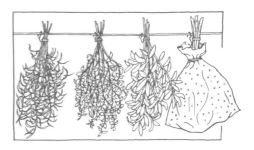

When drying several bunches of herbs on a line, keep them well-spaced.

of the bag. Or you can make quick screens by stapling sheer curtains to a frame. (I use curtains because they are available at nearly every garage sale for a few pennies.) Lay the herbs out in a thin layer to dry. This screen works well for loose blossoms and leaves.

When the herbs are crispy-dry, simply transfer them to airtight containers such as glass jars. If you are a purist, you could make a *muk-kuk,* or birch-bark box. The bark of paper birch has mold-inhibiting agents, which facilitates storage. Two young men once described a food cache they had found while camping in central Wisconsin; being hungry, they ate the food. Later they had an expert look at the handmade containers. He estimated them to be more than five hundred years old. But the food had been edible! Later they found the seeds to be viable, and the herbs potent.

Freezing

If I'm going to use an herb for dinner (dandelion or violet greens) or as a poultice (plantain or comfrey), I prefer to freeze it. Blanch the herb in boiling water for 1 minute. Then drain and immediately plunge the herb into ice water to cool it down. Drain again. To prevent ending up with a quart-size lump of frozen herb, spread the herb in a thin layer on a tray and place it in the freezer to quick-freeze. Transfer it into freezer containers, and take out only as much herb as needed at any one time.

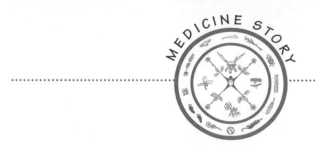

HOW ROSE GOT HER THORNS

When the world was young, Rose had no thorns. Her stems were as smooth as a beetle's shell — and all the animals loved Rose. Rabbit loved Rose. He loved to nibble on her leaves. He could hardly wait until the new spring shoots burst forth. Rose's leaves were best when young and tender.

Deer loved Rose. When the snows were deep, Deer browsed on Rose's twigs. And as the snow melted in the Maple Syrup Moon, Deer browsed Rose to the ground. But Rose was hardy. She grew back from her roots.

Mouse loved Rose. He loved to make his nests in her tangled shelter. He loved her bark. It kept his family fed through the winter. But the shoots that Mouse gnawed on died. Rose grew new shoots, but it took a lot of energy.

Birds loved Rose. They loved to eat the seeds hidden in her fruity hips. They ate a lot to keep strong through the winter. Everyone loved Rose so much that soon there was hardly anything left of her. Her branches were broken, her roots chewed, her flowers fallen, and her seeds gone. She knew she was doomed.

And when Nanaboozhoo (who is the son of the West Wind and a mortal woman) came to visit Rose, he was surprised to see there were no flowers left. Rose cried out, "Won't you help me? They won't let me grow. They are going to kill me!"

Nanaboozhoo went to the animals and begged them to leave Rose be, but the animals hesitated. How could they promise not to eat what was right in front of them or hide where there was shelter? Nanaboozhoo knew the animals were right, but it was clear that Rose's delightful flowers would disappear forever unless he intervened. So he told Rose, "I can't make the animals stop, but maybe I can help you protect yourself." He covered Rose with sharp thorns — everywhere but on her beautiful flowers. This is why Rose has thorns. She reminds us not to love her too well.

I first heard this story told by Margaret Peschel (Keewaydinoquay), an herbal medicine woman from the Leelanau Peninsula in northern Michigan. It is also recorded in Legends of Green Sky Hill by Louise J. Walker. Versions of this story are common among the Anishinaabe peoples of the Three Fires: Ojibway, Ottawa, and Potawatomi.

CHAPTER 2
Selecting Quality
Ingredients and Equipment

It is the ability to choose which makes us human.

— Madelaine L'Engle, *Walking on Water: Reflections on Faith and Art*

An herb's quality determines its healing capacity. Would you eat a salad made from brown wilted lettuce or dried lettuce greens? Certainly not by choice. If it were served in a restaurant you'd demand a refund. Yet we pay for poor-quality herbs wrapped in expensive high quality packages all the time. To ensure that we have the best herbal medicine, we must train ourselves to look beyond the wrapping and into the herb itself.

WHAT MAKES A QUALITY HERB?

Given all possible choices, I *always* choose the fresh herb. The fresh plant has a vitality that quickly degrades. Studies done by the Rodale Institute show that a head of broccoli left out in the sun can lose as much as half of its vitamin C content in the first half hour! In the refrigerator, nutrient loss slows but still occurs. Careful herbalists gather or grow their own herbs whenever possible to ensure the best quality.

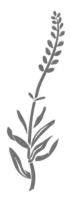

Dried Herbs: Read the Labels

If fresh herbs are unavailable, use dried herbs or products made from certified organic herbs. First try your local county extension office to see who may be growing and selling organic herbs in your area. Or, to purchase retail, look for products stamped with a label from one of the following organic associations whose members have taken a pledge to uphold certain voluntary standards: The Organic Crop Improvement Association (OCIA), Farm-verified Organics, Organic Buyers and Growers Association (OBGA), or the California Certification for Organic Farmers, the latter being regulated by the California state government. As of this writing, there are no *national* guidelines for organic certification, and because of strife between organic growers and the United States Department of Agriculture, there may never be such guidelines.

There are not even any voluntary controls on imported herbs. Pesticides such as DDT that are banned in the United States are routinely used in other nations. In addition, imported herbs must be warehoused for extended periods of time and are routinely fumigated with a toxic soup of chemicals to prevent mold, fungal growth, and insect infestations. Now imagine taking these imported herbs as medicine . . . no thanks. Be particular: About 75 percent of botanicals in medicinal products are imported. Of the remaining 25 percent grown domestically, only a small percentage are certified as organically grown.

Once I find that an herb is certified organic (or ethically wildcrafted) I check the label for a date. Most dried herbs have a shelf life of one year, although some with fleeting essences, such as lemon balm, are only medicinally viable for about six months. Commercial vinegared herbs are considered potent for about one year; tinctures and glycerates for about five years in optimal storage conditions. Heat, light, and air all degrade the quality of the herb. Herbs displayed in clear glass jars in a sunny window have their medicinal virtues compromised. Don't buy them.

> I believe a leaf of grass
> is no less
> Than the journey work
> of the stars.
>
> — Walt Whitman,
> "Song of Myself"

Rely on Your Senses!

If there is no date on the package of dried herbs you're buying — and usually there isn't — take a close look at the herb. The color should be deep and rich, comparable to its living color. Smell it; the odor should be full and strong. The herb itself should be crisp and dry. If you're buying an herb cream, tincture, oil, or other mixture, make sure there is no separation, precipitate, or surface mold. All of these are signs of poor manufacturing or storage.

Be Suspicious of Capsules

Ever notice how you can't check the quality of herb capsules until after you buy them? To test the quality, pour the contents of a purchased herb capsule into a bowl and a bit of a similar dried herb into another bowl for comparison. The whole dried herb will have a stronger smell and color, indicative of a higher quality herb. That's because capsules generally contain the worst-quality herbs commercially available. And even if the manufacturer purchases high-quality herbs to make the capsules, it honestly doesn't matter. The encapsulation process itself ruins the herb.

Have you ever shredded lettuce and let it sit for a couple of hours? It soon wilts, then rots quickly. When an herb is pulverized into powder, the heat generated by the equipment literally cooks the herb. Decay accelerates because more of the herb is exposed to air. Then the encapsulated powder sits decaying further on a shelf for months or years before it's purchased.

When finally ingested, a capsule can take thirty minutes to dissolve, completely bypassing the stomach's digestion and relying on the small intestine for initial breakdown (not the small intestine's best function). You'd probably get a greater medicinal virtue by making a cup of tea from a first-cutting hay bale. A cup of tea made from hay will start to enter the bloodstream before you even swallow. Hay certainly costs a lot less and is usually locally available. And most farmers won't spray a hayfield, since it's not cost-effective. But don't go out and start using hay for medicine — there is one important piece of information about a hay bale you don't know: what plants are inside. The risk of toxic herbs being present is just too great!

Using capsules can give us an herb, but it can never nurture our spirits the way other methods of herb use do. Taking the time to sip a cup of tea or to soak in an herb bath reaffirms the healing process. It helps to slow your pace, empower your being, and delight your senses.

MAKING YOUR OWN CAPSULES

If you have to have your herbs in capsule form for convenience's sake, it's best to make your own. This is best done by grinding the herb by hand with a mortar and pestle, since a mechanical grinder generates too much heat. Make only one or two days' supply at a time, and refrigerate the capsules until used.

GOOD MEDICINE STARTS WITH GOOD INGREDIENTS

In addition to herbs, there are a number of other ingredients we are going to need for creating our own homemade remedies. As a self-reliant herbalist, I want these additional ingredients to be of as high a quality as the herbs I use. Let the large mass-manufacturer of lip balm use less expensive paraffin wax instead of beeswax. For my purposes, the extra half penny per ounce that beeswax costs is well worth the difference on my baby's chapped bottom.

A Guide to Quality

There are several basic ingredients you'll be using over and over again for the recipes in this book. Following is a description of these ingredients, along with advice on how to ensure purity and the highest quality for each.

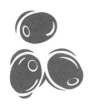

OILS
Oils exposed to light and heat quickly become rancid, and rancid oils are carcinogenic. If an oil is in a clear bottle, glass or plastic, it may well be rancid. It's important to ask the store owner how long the oil has been sitting on the shelf. An owner who is confident about the quality of the oils may let you sample. One quick way to test for rancidity is to put a drop of oil on the back of your tongue: If it burns, it is rancid. Another good policy is to purchase medicinal oils that are packaged in tins or dark bottles. Be sure that any oils you buy are cold-pressed; any other extraction process uses chemical solvents to increase the oil yield.

Internal use. My oil of choice for internal consumption is olive oil. It is readily available in tins, is quality graded, and tastes delicious. Olive oil is also rich in antioxidants, which are food compounds (such as the vitamins A, C, and E and carotenes and selenium) that combat destructive free oxygen molecules. Antioxidants thus help the body fight degenerative and age-related illnesses. Adding an herb such as ginger to the olive oil allows it to do double duty as a healing oil and a base for cooking, saving a little work. When colds are coming on in our family, I will often sauté a little gingerroot or other warming herb in the olive oil I am using to make dinner. That way we can have our medicine and eat it too.

In selecting olive oil, you should know that it is graded: The first cold-pressing yields the highest grade, extra virgin, which is best for internal uses. Organically grown cold-pressed canola oil makes a less expensive substitute. When I'm on a budget, I mix equal amounts of olive oil and canola oil, with satisfactory results.

External use (absorption). As an external absorption oil used to soften, moisturize, and maintain healthy skin, I prefer to use jojoba oil (which technically is a plant ester, not an oil). It is readily absorbed by the skin and resists rancidity. It is priced competitively with other absorbing oils such as sesame, walnut, wheat germ, and safflower. Unlike these oils, however, jojoba oil should not be used internally.

External use (nonabsorbent). For a nonabsorbent oil (for massages, chapped skin, diaper rash), use one that forms a protective barrier on the skin. Oils that are not absorbed as easily and are pleasant to work with include sweet almond, virgin olive, avocado, peanut, apricot kernel, and cocoa butter.

ALCOHOLS

Alcohols are primarily used to make tinctures. The concentration of alcohol is usually expressed as a percentage; multiply the percentage by 2 to get what is called the proof. Thus 80-proof vodka is 40 percent alcohol. Any 80-proof alcohol will make an acceptable tincture for most herbs. If 190-proof (95 percent alcohol, also known as everclear or grain alcohol) is legally available in your area, I recommend using it instead. Using 190-proof offers several advantages over lower-proof alcohol:

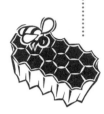

- ◆ Less is required per dose.
- ◆ With grain alcohol I can easily control the amount of water I add. The alcohol extracts the herb by desiccation, essentially wringing out the aromatic essences of the herb into the alcohol. Some herbs, such as ginger, need the stronger concentration of alcohol because some of its medicinal compounds are not fully solvent in water. Some herbs (most flowers and leaves) need more water.
- ◆ It has a longer shelf life.
- ◆ Because of the further distillation, the alcohol is less likely to have wayside contaminants or flavoring agents added.

WINES

Don't use commercial wines for medicine making. Wine grapes are heavily sprayed with fungal and mold inhibitors, and sulfites and cadmium are used to make the wine. Studies have also shown that the foil wrapper around the seal leaks lead into the wine. But don't rule out medicinal wines altogether; chapter 6 includes recipes for simple, low-cost medicinal wines you can make at home.

VINEGARS

A good-quality vinegar is alive. Vinegar is made by inoculating wine with bacteria (called the mother vinegar). A living vinegar is slightly cloudy, and there is a sediment on the bottom of the bottle. You can buy apple cider vinegar with the mother in it at most health food stores, but it is a bit pricey. Chapter 6 includes instructions for making your own vinegar for a few pennies a gallon.

GLYCERIN

Glycerin is used to make tinctures for children or adults who wish to avoid alcohol. Glycerin's sweetness helps mask unpleasant flavors. Use a 100-percent-vegetable-based glycerin; the quality is higher than animal-based glycerin and is safe for human consumption. The shelf life is comparable to that of alcohol tinctures, though glycerin does not extract resins or oils from plants well.

Glycerin should be diluted with water when making the tincture (the same as alcohol, but remember, many alcohols are purchased diluted). Use pure distilled water to ensure no wayside contaminants. A tincture made with glycerin is called a glycerate. Excessive consumption of glycerate tinctures may cause diarrhea in sensitive indiviudals. (See page 48 for standard tincture doses.)

HONEY

Buy honey that is free of pesticides and contaminants. By and large I find that small beekeepers avoid using sprays — perhaps because beekeeping by its very nature involves an understanding of nature's web. Try to buy honey grown close to your home. Each country — indeed, each county — produces a distinct type of honey. People with hay fever or allergies sometimes find relief from eating local honey. Stop at your local farmer's market, and find a person who is selling crystallized honey. This honey is raw and unfiltered. Raw honey contains enzymes that have antibiotic abilities — enzymes that are destroyed by light and heat, making raw honey the best choice for medicinal use. I think it tastes better as well. There are people who swear by the superior qualities of dark honey; however, medicinally I find little difference between the two.

CAUTION

The Centers for Disease Control in Atlanta recommends that raw honey should not be given to children under one year old. You may wish to play it safe and avoid giving honey to children for their first two years. Some uncooked honeys may contain botulism spores that are harmless for the older child and adult, but can cause a fatal diarrhea in an immature digestive system.

BEESWAX

Try to buy your beeswax from a local beekeeper. You'll get a better-quality wax for a much lower price. The beekeeper I get wax from charges me $6 per pound; the local craft store charges $2.50 per ounce! Don't worry if there are a few bee wings or such in the wax. Wax acts as a preservative, and you can simply strain out the stray pieces when you melt it.

SUGARS

Sugars are used to make wines and syrups, and to sweeten bitter brews. Alternatives to refined white table sugar include honey (see above) and maple syrup. Maple syrup contains trace minerals that are carried up in a tree's sap from as much as 60 feet below the ground. A pure maple syrup has a flowery aroma and buttery texture. Grade A Amber syrup comes from the first flow of sap and is considered the best.

Stevia. This herbal sweetener has been used worldwide for centuries, but has been available in the United States only since 1988. The Food and Drug Administration has not approved stevia as a sweetener, only as a food additive. It's up to three hundred times sweeter than sugar; use just 1 teaspoon of stevia in place of 1 cup of sugar. Its sweetening ability is similar to that of sucrose, with little aftertaste. Stevia has a fleeting flavor, reminiscent of honeysuckle, that seems to disappear in tea or cooking. Another plus is that stevia is not a nutrition source for oral bacteria; it actually helps suppress cavities!

SALTS

Salts are effective for preserving herbs to be used in baths. Common table salt, sodium chloride, is generally not recommended, but will do if no other salt is available. Sea salt, refined from ocean brine and rich in minerals, is my preference. Epsom salt, also known as magnesium sulfate, is an inexpensive alternative when you're making bath salts.

BASIC EQUIPMENT: AS CLOSE AS YOUR KITCHEN

The equipment you use to make your remedies will affect how they turn out. The good news is that home herbalism requires no special distillers, tubes, condensers, or other supplies. Chances are you have everything you need already — or you can find it at a garage sale for next to nothing.

NOTEBOOK

A blank notebook is your most important piece of equipment. Be sure to keep track of your favorite recipes, references, and suppliers' addresses and telephone numbers. Because I gather or grow nearly all my herbs, I also note the seasonal and daily weather conditions, gathering dates and places. I write notes and observations about the preparation process. I even write down my mistakes — they are valuable little lessons that I don't wish to repeat.

LABELS

However large or small, fancy or plain, labels are the herbalist's best friend. Use them relentlessly; a remedy is not finished until it has a label on it. At the very least, list the ingredients and the date. Other helpful items to list are: what the preparation is for, how it should be used, how it should be stored, and where the herbs were obtained.

GLASS JARS

Colored glass jars and bottles with lids are treasures to any herbalist. Check out your local recycling station for free jars. A local restaurant-bar lets me haul away as many empty liquor and wine bottles and 1-gallon-size pickle jars as I care to — Saturday night offers me the best selection. Second-hand shops always offer interesting selections, usually for less than a dime apiece. Disinfect the bottles before using by boiling for 10 minutes, or rinse with a 3 percent hydrogen peroxide solution, commonly available at a

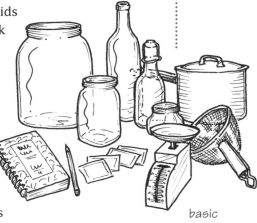

basic equipment

grocery store or pharmacy. Simply wash your jars with soap and water and rinse. Then, pour a small amount of peroxide into the jar, shake vigorously, and drain. Last, rinse with water and air dry.

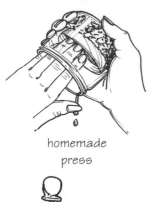

homemade
press

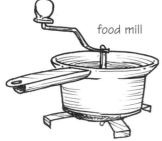

food mill

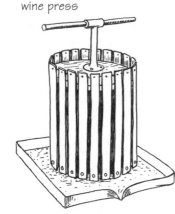

wine press

STRAINER AND PRESS

To strain a cup of tea, any stainless-steel sieve works well. But you might notice that, when you strain, you're losing a lot of precious liquid from the loose herbs — that's valuable medicine. Likewise, when we talk about casually tossing out the spent herbs used to make a jojoba herb oil or a carefully compiled tincture, suddenly every drop that can be pressed from them becomes precious. A press works much better than a strainer for these purposes.

A quick and effective homemade press can be assembled simply from a lid that fits inside your jar. Apply wrist pressure to the lid to squeeze out as much liquid extract as possible. I have used a food mill (the kind used to strain baby food) with more satisfying results. But for the best extraction, it is hard to beat a wine press. This piece of equipment is common, inexpensive, and easy to use. You can find one at most kitchen accessory stores or beer and wine-making suppliers. Do tell them that you are using it only for home herb use lest they try to sell you a commercial grape crusher!

MORTAR AND PESTLE

If you're only going to buy one piece of special equipment for making herbal remedies, this is it. A mortar and pestle for grinding dried roots, leaves, and seeds is the only way to be assured of a fresh herb powder. A traditional European mortar has smooth sides. A Japanese mortar, called a *suribachi,* has grooves and ridges on the sides; I find this style to be more efficient. If you live near a flowing creek, you can look to any little waterfalls for natural stone mortars made of quartz or basalt. I have a 2-foot stone slab that I use as my mortar, along with fist-size round rocks for my pestles for extra-quick grinding.

Herbs can also be ground efficiently in a hand-cranked coffee grinder set aside just for herbs. (Don't use it to make coffee afterward, or your coffee will taste like the herbs.) And even though electric coffee grinders may seem more efficient, try to avoid them. The herbs get too hot, which destroys delicate oils and essences. If you need the ease of an electric grinder, some experienced medicine makers freeze the herbs first to keep temperatures to a minimum. Grind small batches using only short bursts and you can keep the herbs from getting hot.

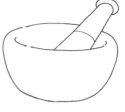

mortar and pestle

SAUCEPAN

Reserve one 1- or 2-quart pan just for making salves. Oils and beeswax leave hard-to-clean residues behind in the pan. It only took one batch of waxy chicken soup to convince me that a separate salve pan was a wise investment. Similarly, reserve one stainless steel or birch stirring spoon and one stainless steel mesh strainer that fits over your saucepan for salve making.

SCALE

A small diet scale is a useful piece of equipment to have on hand for making herbal remedies, since weight is a more precise unit of measure than volume. For most mild herbs, the medicinal dose is 1 ounce of herb to 32 ounces of water. Because an ounce of dried leaves has greater volume than an ounce of root, most beginners find it helpful to use a scale until they become accustomed to the proportions.

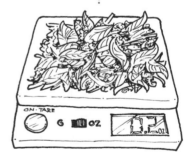

scale

However I never did use a scale for making medicine with mild herbs until I began to teach others. I reasoned that since the herbs were relatively safe, exploring the differences in taste and potency was more important to me than obtaining a precise measurement. And since an herb's relative strength depends on so many variables, it isn't possible to measure potency anyway — unless you have equipment far more sophisticated than a simple scale. Still, when you're starting out, a scale will help you get a feel for the relative suggested proportions.

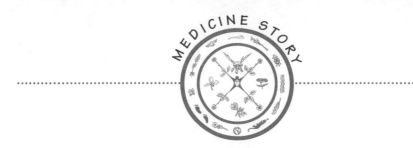

HOW TO FIND A LOST ARROW — OR ANYTHING ELSE

One day a young boy was playing with his toy arrows, and one by one broke all of them. He wanted to keep playing, so he went and took one of his father's arrows. Now, all a man owns is his bow and arrows and clothes; everything else — the wigwam, the skins, the food, even the children — belongs to the women. Each man's arrows are treasured and many hours are spent crafting them and making them perfect. They protect, provide his people with meat, and give him honor. This boy must have been young indeed not to remember this when he took his father's arrow.

All the boy knew was how well his shots flew — farther and faster than ever. Once, the arrow went so far that he lost sight of it. But he was able to mark the arrow's flight and ran over to seek it in the place he had spotted. To his dismay, the area was a muddy overgrown tangle. He climbed a nearby tree to peer in, but he couldn't see the arrow anywhere. So he plunged into the thicket to look. He knew he'd better find that arrow!

His first steps covered his moccasins with mud. He searched and he searched, but he couldn't find the arrow. He kept worrying about what his father would say or do to him, until he made himself scared. He looked till he was tired, and hot, and frustrated. It wasn't until he felt itchy all over that he finally noticed where he really was — right in the middle of a poison ivy patch! Now he was in big trouble! His father was going to be furious, and his mother, too! No one could help him. Overwhelmed, the boy sat down and began to bawl.

Through his tears, he noticed a frog jump near his feet. "You're in big trouble too, frog," he said out loud. "Don't you know you'll get poison ivy all over your smooth skin, just like me?" The frog stared at him, jumped over to some broad-leafed plants, and rubbed his body against the leaves. Then he stuck out his tongue and jumped away.

So the boy gathered up some of those same leaves and rubbed himself, too. And as he stooped down to gather some more, he saw his father's arrow under the leaves. He picked it up and cleaned off the mud. He left behind a pinch of tobacco to thank the frog — and, I'm told, he even remembered to clean his moccasins!

Versions of this story are common among the Anishinaabe peoples of the northern Great Lakes region. The plant used in the story could be plantain, curly dock, or jewelweed. All grow near poison ivy, and each is effective against it.

CHAPTER 3
Making a Simple Cup of Tea

*Simplicity is the final flower; behind it are cataclysms
of the soul and accumulations of wisdom,
just as behind the simplicity of a leaf are cosmic
and geological changes without number.*

— Claude Bragdon, *The New Image,* 1928

Ever since some ingenious cavewoman threw a handful of wild herbs in her family's water-skin to keep the water tasting fresh and wholesome, herbal medicine has been with us — arguably the world's oldest science. Every single culture in the world steeps herbs in water for refreshing and medicinal drinks. Every single one.

Herbal medicine seems amazingly complex at first. There are over ten thousand plants listed in the collective written worldwide pharmacopeias! But just as nature has the salmon lay ten thousand eggs so that one might survive to adulthood, she has given us ten thousand plants to ensure that one will be available when we need it. A question I am often asked is, "What herb shall I take for my illness?" I like to answer, "Take any herb — just be sure it's a simple one!"

It's best to pick one or two plants that you are already familiar with and explore them fully. Only after you gain confidence in using those plants in teas, poultices, salves, or tinctures should you move on to learn about another plant. Let yourself build a basic foundation of knowledge from which one day you'll feel confident enough to dive into the whole pool of herbal medicine.

THE ART OF SIMPLING

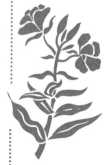

Herbal medicine can be so easy that it's simple. In fact, it's even called simpling. But don't let the name fool you into thinking that simpling isn't as effective as more complex formulas. To the contrary, simpling is the recommended course of treatment for most common acute ailments.

Four Elements

Successful simpling involves four elements or principles. First, you must use mild plants. These are often the plants commonly used as foods. They are safe enough for small children and the elderly, enhance the body's capacity to heal itself, and help create long-term health.

Second, you must use these mild herbs in large doses. The cup of tea you make from a paper tea bag may taste nice, but its medicinal action is negligible. Simpling involves making a strong pot of tea and drinking it several times throughout the day — for days, weeks, and sometimes months until a satisfactory cure is seen. For some chronic illnesses, such as diabetes, the simple herbs may become a lifelong habit.

The third element of simpling is that you must use herbs that grow nearby. The practical reason for this is purely economic. At three to ten dollars per ounce, you could easily spend upward of three hundred dollars a month for an herbal remedy. But more important, herbs take on the characteristics of their habitat. Just as herbs growing in wet places swell with water and therefore work better for kidney and bladder ailments, so herbs growing in cold climates tend to be more building and warming, and herbs grown in hot climates tend to be more eliminating and cooling.

To a certain extent, each climate tends to breed particular types of ailments in the people who live there. It is no surprise that you find more parasitic diseases in hotter climates, and more respiratory ailments in colder climates. By using the plants that grow in your own region, you are turning to the herbs that are best adapted for the stresses your climate puts on your body.

The fourth, and most important, element of simpling is that you must be patiently committed to following the course of the cure. It takes time to gather herbs

---

FOUR ELEMENTS OF SIMPLING

1. Use mild herbs.
2. Use the herbs in large doses.
3. Use herbs that grow in or near the area where you live.
4. Be patient and committed to waiting for the effects of the tea you make.

and make a simple tea, and it takes responsibility to drink that tea for several days or weeks as required. Usually, however, you should see some measure of relief within two to three days. If not, consider trying a different herb. When you use an herb for an extended period of time, take a rest from it one or two days a week, to give your body a chance to regain equilibrium.

For true healing to begin, you must also address other factors affecting health, such as stress, poor diet, exposure to toxins, and emotional or spiritual discontent. Lao-tzu said it well in his *Tao Te Ching:* "A person will get well only when he is tired of being sick."

HOW TO MAKE A SIMPLE TEA

The purpose of making a cup of tea is to extract the medicinal virtues of an herb into a cup of water. If you keep that in mind, the process becomes easy, and terms such as *decoction, infusion* (which are preparation techniques), *poultice, plaster,* and *fomentation* (application techniques) become unimportant. As you gain experience working with the herbs, methods of process and application do become important. But don't get hung up on definitions so much that you prevent yourself from exploring the herbs in the first place. Remember the intent is simply to make a cup of tea; the rest will follow.

The Method for Delicate Leaves and Flowers

Begin with 1 ounce of dried herb or 2 ounces of fresh herb; bring 1 quart of water to just under the boiling point, and pour it over the herb. Let sit for about 20 minutes, or until the water has absorbed the fragrance and color of the herb. This recipe will yield about 3 cups, which is one day's dose, taken ½ cup at a time through the day.

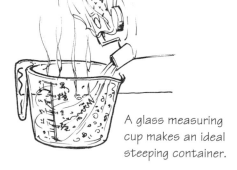

A glass measuring cup makes an ideal steeping container.

Alternate method. Another common method of simpling with flowers and leaves is to put the herb in cold water and let it sit in the sun for several hours. You can also put the herb in cold water and let it sit for 24 hours in the refrigerator. This method is preferred for herbs that have heat-sensitive volatile oils you want to preserve, such as mint and rose petal. It usually extracts the greatest amount of minerals from the herbs, but a lesser amount of tannins (which give herbs such as rose petal and blackberry their astringency).

The Method for Hardy Roots, Seeds, and Barks

It takes more effort to chew a root than to chew a leaf, and it takes more energy to extract the virtues from roots, seeds, and barks than from leaves or flowers. Grind, mash, or cut the herb first so as to expose more of its surface area to the water, making the extraction process more complete.

Measure 1 ounce of dried herb or 2 ounces fresh herb and combine in a saucepan with 1 quart of water. Simmer over low heat for 20 minutes to 1 hour. Herbs with important volatile oils, such as burdock, ginger, and mullein root, should be kept covered. For herbs left uncovered, a simple guideline is to simmer until the water is reduced by about one-third. This recipe yields 1 to 2 cups of tea, the daily dose, which is best drunk in small sips throughout the day.

Alternate method. Another method I like is making a sun tea. Begin by pouring 1 quart of boiling water over the cut or chopped herb. Put out in the sun and allow to sit for a full day. This process generally extracts less of an herb's medicinal attributes but keeps more of its vitamins and nutritive integrity.

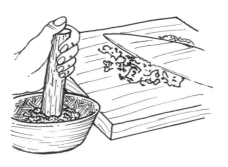

Mash or chop the hardy roots, seeds, and barks of herbs to prepare them for making tea.

WATER IS MEDICINE, TOO!

Water is a powerful healing ally. Considered the blood of the mother earth, water helps focus and direct nature's forces. It has the capacity to absorb and reflect back energy — both measurable physical energies such as light, elements, and chemicals, and any intangible emotional or spiritual energies you may place into the water. Always make your tea with the best possible water available.

SELECTING HERBS: START WITH WHAT YOU KNOW

As Maria Von Trapp said, "It's always best to start at the beginning." Look about you. What plants are you familiar with? Can you recognize a dandelion? A white pine tree? A strawberry? Now ask yourself what you have access to and make a list. These are the plants you should choose from for your teas. Just be sure to research the herb's safeness for consumption before you begin gathering.

Using Different Parts of the Plant

One of the gifts of herbalism is that one plant can yield us many medicines, depending on which part of the plant is used. As you work with an herb, explore its different parts. We know the strawberry best for its delicious fruit. However, the leaves, blossoms, stems, and roots all have valuable and different medicinal virtues — which vary further depending on when you gather them. Again, research the plant before you use it. For example, while rhubarb stalks are edible, rhubarb leaves can be poisonous. In the list that follows, you will find details about which parts of twenty-five plants are most commonly used.

WARNING: RESEARCH PLANTS FIRST

Always research any plant before you decide to make a tea from it. Just because a plant or herb is familiar doesn't mean it is safe. Nutmeg is commonly found in most kitchens, for instance, but is toxic in relatively small doses. So keep a good herbal medicine reference book on hand (see Home Remedy Library on page 156) to use before you sip.

TWENTY-FIVE SIMPLE HERBS
TO KNOW AND USE

The plants described on the following pages are a selection of perennial favorites for beginning students of herbalism. They are common, easy to recognize and gather, safe, and fun to work with. I encourage you to branch out and explore other plants as well.

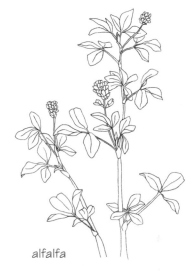
alfalfa

ALFALFA *(MEDICAGO SATIVA)*
The Arabic word for *alfalfa* means "father," and the plant was once reserved for warriors and prized horses. It's a superlative restorative tonic. Use the whole flowering plant for digestive weakness, for chronic inflammations, and to rebuild vitality. Deep taproots enable alfalfa to bring many trace minerals into its leaves, as well as vitamins C, D, E, and K. Though the roots aren't often used, I find that they make an excellent wash for chronic skin disorders.

BLACKBERRY (*RUBUS* SPP.)
To find the best stands of blackberry, look for their showy flowers in the spring. Blackberry root combats the deadly dysentery that runs rampant in close-quartered camps. In the American

---

ONE MAN'S MEAT IS ANOTHER MAN'S POISON

When trying a new plant, there is always the possibility of individual allergic reaction. Simple and mild herbs generally are safe to test at home. First, rub a bit of the plant on a patch of skin. If no swelling or itching occurs in 24 hours, try drinking a small amount of tea made from that herb. Wait 24 hours before taking a larger dose.

Some people find themselves allergic to many members of a whole family of plants. For example, people who are allergic to strawberry may have a similar reaction to rose hips or raspberry; all are members of the rose family of plants.

Revolutionary War, both sides accepted truces to enable the troops to "go rooting." The leaves are milder. Blackberry root (use for adults) or leaves (use for children) is still one of the safest and surest remedies for diarrhea. I make a blackberry root vinegar that excels at alleviating diarrhea caused both by flu or mild food poisoning. The flowers have a gentle sweetness that add a pleasant dimension to tea blends. And, of course, the fruits aren't so bad either.

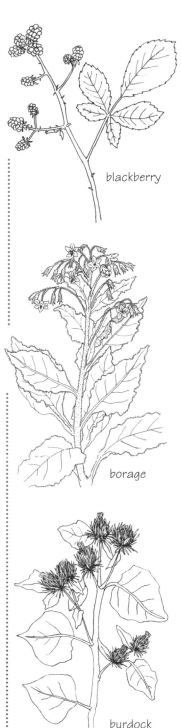

blackberry

BORAGE (BORAGO OFFICINALIS)

I only had to plant borage once — it volunteered thereafter. Borage's delicate blue flowers make salads and teas festive; they can also be added to homemade wine. The leaf, which has a cooling cucumber flavor, reduces fevers and calms irritated tissues. A glass of cold borage lemonade is one of the most refreshing summer drinks I know of; served hot it soothes a sore throat. The newly emerging leaves are a pleasant nibble, but as they grow they quickly get too prickly to eat. Having been a nursing mother of twins, I can assure you that borage ensures even milk production and high energy levels. Throughout history, borage has helped invalids regain their strength, and it works just as well today.

The seed oil extract improves adrenal function, easing the stresses of menopause, obesity, rheumatism, and steroid or antibiotic treatments.

borage

BURDOCK (ARCTIUM LAPPA)

Nature's Velcro and the original dart, burdock is one of the best tonic herbs — bar none. Use all parts; the seed and root are the most effective, however. Use the seeds externally for skin eruptions, while simultaneously using the root internally to treat the cause.

Burdock is used to eliminate toxins in the body. The root promotes sweating, increases

burdock

urine output, enhances liver function, and tastes very good in stir-fries, or slow-roasted or grilled. The peeled first-year stalk is another yummy food, similar to celery. The seeds are antibacterial and anti-inflammatory.

CATNIP *(NEPETA CATARIA)*

One of my first herbs of choice for children, nursing mothers, and the elderly, catnip calms the nerves, soothes digestion, and lowers a fever without raising it first. I've also used it successfully to ease colic, calm gastric and duodenal ulcers, aid digestion, increase milk flow, ease stress, and torment my cat.

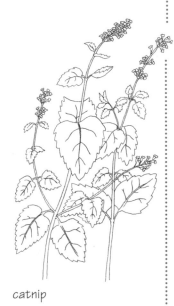

catnip

DANDELION *(TARAXACUM OFFICINALE)*

If you think you've never used dandelion as medicine, guess again. It's a prime ingredient in over half of all herb blends on the market, including formulas for weight loss, PMS, detoxification, and rejuvenation along with liver, digestive, kidney, and skin ailments! Dandelion is such a wondrous source of minerals, vitamins, fiber, micronutrients, lecithin, and biologically active substances that there is probably no existing condition that would not benefit from regularly consuming dandelions.

The greatest gift of dandelion is its safety record. Dandelion has no known cautionary drug interactions, cumulative toxic effects, or contraindications for use. This is one herb to allow yourself the full range of freedom to explore!

All parts are edible. The flowers make pleasant tea and wine, fritters and seasoning. The root can be steamed, broiled, roasted, and toasted for coffee. Eaten with bread, the bitterness in the leaf vanishes. I always use dandelions as food first.

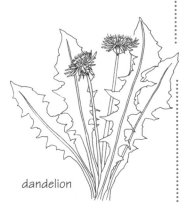

dandelion

For medicine, gather the root in the fall. Employed as a diuretic, dandelion has ample potassium to replace what is lost from frequent urination. Dandelion stimulates liver function, reduces cholesterol, fights diabetes, and stimulates digestion; extracts indicate tumor-fighting capacities on lab-induced breast cancers in mice.

GARLIC *(ALLIUM SATIVUM)*

Even orthodox medicine acknowledges that garlic reduces cholesterol, lowers blood pressure, and decreases the risk of heart attack. But garlic also helps regulate blood sugar levels, is useful in all manner of lung ailments, kills parasites, calms spasms, and relieves inflammation. Did I say it's one of nature's best antibiotic and antiviral agents?

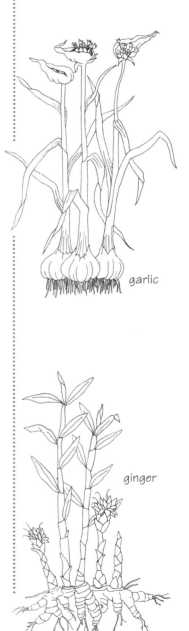

garlic

This is the stuff that daily medicine is made of. For greatest benefits, garlic should be eaten *raw*. Unfortunately, some people cannot tolerate raw garlic on an empty stomach. They could try eating it with bread, or taking a garlic footbath. Garlic will retain some of its cardiovascular benefits when cooked, but heat destroys its antibacterial and antiviral qualities. One clove a day is adequate for preventative purposes. Take more for acute ailments such as colds and flus. For external use, always put garlic on a piece of gauze, then lay the gauze next to the skin; otherwise blistering may occur.

GINGER *(ZINGIBER OFFICINALE)*

Ginger grows outdoors in the southern United States. The rest of us can grow ginger as a houseplant. It likes ample humidity, good light, and about a month to sprout from a root cutting. A classic remedy for colds, flu, fevers, nausea, menstrual cramps, motion sickness, and hangover, ginger stimulates the circulatory system and acts as a general mild stimulant. To bring heat to a specific area, use a compress of ginger. I use it extensively in food, salves, teas, and baths all through the cold months of autumn and winter.

ginger

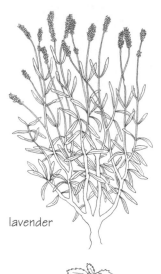

lavender

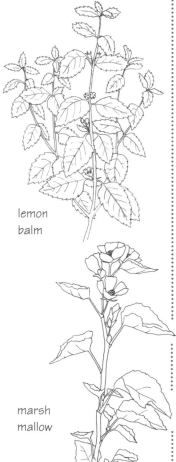

lemon
balm

marsh
mallow

LAVENDER (*LAVANDULA ANGUSTIFOLIA SPP.*)

A voluptuous herb, lavender envelops the senses as she heals. Her scent soothes tension, repels insects, and stimulates penile erection. For medicine, gather the flowers when the petals begin to fade. Their uplifting influence calms jittery nerves, relieves headaches, stimulates appetite, and soothes colic. Use the herb freely in baths, compresses, and salves, or in wines, cooking, baking, and beverages.

LEMON BALM *(MELISSA OFFICINALIS)*

Heed this plant's lemony scent: If there's little aroma, there's little medicine. Fresh is best. Lemon balm brings comfort against despair and melancholy. And since illness always brings a measure of sadness, I turn to this herb to heal both spirit and body. Medicinally, the leaves are cooling: They reduce fevers, soothe bruises and aches, heal wounds, calm nervous stomachs, and help heal sores from herpes viruses.

MARSH MALLOW (*ALTHAEA OFFICINALIS* OR *MALVA SYLVESTRIS* SPP.)

Marsh mallow (and to a lesser degree common garden mallow and hollyhocks) soothes irritated mucous membranes throughout the body. It's successful against all manner of digestive disturbances, sore throats, colds, and coughs. It gives a slippery feel to wines and vinegars without altering the taste. The flower petals are a pleasant nibble, but try those little green cheeses where the seeds are made — they are fun!

MULLEIN *(VERBASCUM THAPSUS)*

With mullein, intent is everything: It's used to make magic and to protect from magic. Each part of mullein contains unique medicine. The flowers kill bacteria, and the infused flower oil soothes wounds and earaches.

You can smoke the leaf to open and relax bronchial passages. It is effective against whooping cough, asthma, and bronchitis. Although the whole plant is sedative, the root concentrates this quality. A boiled root tea calms the body inside and out. *Warning:* Mullein seeds are toxic and should never be used for any reason.

OATS *(AVENA SATIVA)*

Think of oats as a one-penny moisturizer. Tie a handful of rolled oats in a muslin bag. Moisten the bag and rub it on chapped skin, mild sunburn, eczema, insect bites, and itchy rashes — or toss it into a warm bath. This same soluble gummy fiber soothes the intestinal tract and lowers cholesterol. Eat oat porridge during convalescence to rebuild strength. Both the grain and the oat straw nourish nerve cells and help the body cope with insomnia, anxiety, and nerve disorders such as shingles.

PEPPERMINT, SPEARMINT *(MENTHA X PIPERITA, M. SPICATA SPP.)*

There are many varieties of mints, but peppermint and spearmint are the most popular. I use the milder variety, spearmint, for children. Both are cooling, stimulating, and refreshing in action and flavor. I consider mint a summer herb, as a cup of strong tea will bring on a good sweat and cool the body by evaporation. Slightly antiseptic, mint makes a good mouthwash, wound wash, and sore throat remedy. A simple tea is classic for headache and sinus relief. Ever wonder at the tradition of a complimentary mint at the end of a meal? Mint stimulates digestion and relieves nausea — it helps dispel that overfull feeling and possible indigestion or gas.

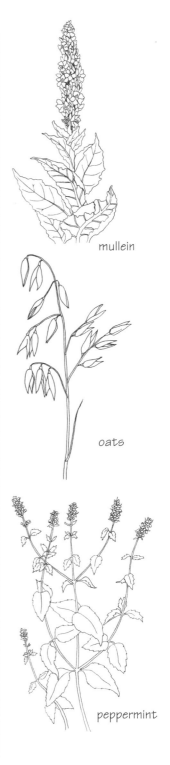

mullein

oats

peppermint

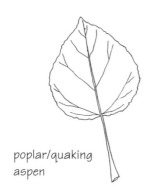

plantain

poplar/quaking
aspen

PLANTAIN (*PLANTAGO MAJOR* SPP., *P. LANCEOLATA* SPP.)

Plantain has followed in mankind's footsteps throughout the world. Perhaps this is a good thing, considering how useful it is. Plantain is a soothing and drawing herb. The leaf is helpful for all manner of external skin irritations and irritations of the digestive system. The seeds are nutritious — they're full of easily assimilated B vitamins. I sprout them throughout the winter months. Used with the husks left on, they are a safe and gentle laxative. The root is an excellent topical dressing to heal stubborn sores. Also known as poor man's spinach, the young leaves may be cut back and lightly steamed. The plant easily grows back from a generous root system, providing you with greens through the summer with no effort other than the harvest.

POPLAR AND/OR QUAKING ASPEN (*POPULUS* SPP.)

Considered a standard remedy in the north woods, this tree grows in dense stands that benefit from being selectively thinned when they are thumb-size saplings. The strongest medicine lies in the inner bark of the trunk. A bitter remedy, poplar contains a substance related to the active ingredient in aspirin (and willow). However, it doesn't irritate the stomach in the same way that refined aspirin will. (**Caution:** As with aspirin, poplar should *not* be taken by children with a high fever.) Poplar buds help break up congestion of the lungs, and aid digestion. They are an old-time remedy for rheumatism, headache, inflamed prostate, and general weakness. A salve made from the sticky buds makes a good deep muscle rub. Make a tincture with the buds of balsam poplar for a natural preservative similar to its commercial counterpart, tincture of benzoin.

RASPBERRY *(RUBUS IDAEUS)*

This is the woman's herb. Drink tea made from the second year's leaf growth to prepare for an easy childbirth and prevent miscarriage. Less astringent and safer for children than its relative the blackberry, raspberry relieves diarrhea and skin irritations. Since the taste of the leaf is somewhat harsh (I like it, though), leaves are seldom used alone, but are the prime ingredient in many herbal formulas. The fruit is a nourishing tonic as well as a gourmet treat. Slightly wilted raspberry leaves may have toxic properties, so be sure to use them fresh or completely dried.

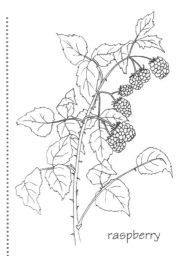

raspberry

CAUTION

Improperly dried leaves of raspberry, strawberry, blackberry, and sweet clovers may contain a compound produced from residual moisture and fungal activity that inhibits blood clotting and may cause internal hemmorraging. Be sure to use these herb leaves fresh or completely dried only. Some herbalists recommend avoiding them altogether (especially red clover) for several weeks prior to surgical procedures or childbirth.

RED CLOVER *(TRIFOLIUM PRATENSE)*

This was the first plant I let myself "play" with. I tried red clover tea, hair rinse, foot powder, and jelly. I used it for colds and colic, in soups, cakes, cookies, and wine. Finally, I developed a feel for red clover. Don't let the following suggestions limit your "play" with red clover.

Red clover is slightly sweet and cooling. The fresh flowers provide relief from minor inflammations. Internally, red clover rebuilds the body's strength from chronic disorders such as allergies and arthritis. It's been shown to be

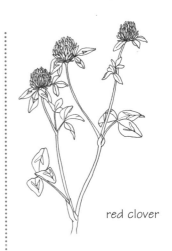

red clover

effective against chemotherapy's side effects. Drunk consistently over a long period of time, it reduces the blood's ability to clot, and while many people have found this herb helps them combat arteriosclerosis, it could prove dangerous during surgery or childbirth. It is wise to remember to take one or two days' rest a week from this herb to help give the body a chance to return to balance, and to avoid it during the last month of pregnancy or before surgery. Gather flowers before they're fully open.

ROSE (*ROSA RUGOSA* SPP.)

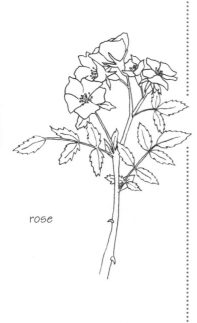

rose

Old-fashioned roses make the best medicines; avoid using hybrid roses. Roses are sweet, astringent, and lightly cooling in medicinal action. Gather the petals before the flower is pollinated, from the flowers that have a bright sunny yellow center. They have not been pollinated yet and are producing a scent to call to the bees. After pollination, the center anthers turn brown and dry up. The scent is noticeably weaker; soon the petals will fade and drop. Rose petals added to your medicinal preparations will impart a pleasant flavor. To use externally, gather the leaves before the flower buds appear. The petals bring delight to the senses, lighten the spirits, and are mildly astringent. The hips are full of vitamin C, and best gathered after a hard frost. Hidden within the seeds is a storehouse of vitamin E. The whole hips were traditionally set by for late winter to use as a blood purifier.

ST.-JOHN'S-WORT *(HYPERICUM PERFORATUM)*

St.-John's-wort

This herb's action is specific to the nervous system. Use it topically to relieve neuralgia or back pain, or to heal cleaned wounds quickly. Drinking the tea calms nervous tension — it can even ease clinical depression — and gives the body an anti-viral boost. Look carefully at a leaf and you'll see tiny black dots. This is where the medicine lies. About a week after the flowering, pick a blossom and rub it on your palm. If it leaves red-purple streaks behind, the plant is ready to gather. Gather the top quarter of the whole plant. Some people become sensitive to sunlight after drinking the tea for extended periods of time.

STRAWBERRY (*FRAGARIA VESCA* SPP.)

Strawberry teaches us to pay attention to gathering times. All parts are medicinal, and the medicinal virtue of each part changes throughout the growing season. For example, the unopened blossom is somewhat bitter and astringent, useful against diarrhea and upset stomach. The fully opened flower is fragrant and sweet and stimulates appetite. The stalk in early spring is a tasty nibble; in midsummer it stanches bleeding from a cut. The overall balanced mineral content of strawberry leaf tones the heart and blood vessels. But I'll allow you to discover for yourself when it's best to gather.

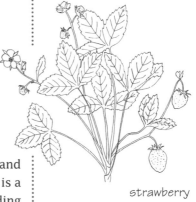

strawberry

THYME (*THYMUS VULGARIS* SPP.)

Modern medicine may have little to offer you against viral infections — but herbalists have thyme. Drink thyme at the onset of a cold or chills to increase the efficiency of the immune system. The tea is also antimicrobial, antifungal, and mildly styptic, making it excellent for external cuts and wounds. Thyme tea warms the stomach, eases cramps, and calms nervous conditions. The plant is so useful that it is known as mother of thyme, or mother's thyme! Avoid frequent large doses of thyme during the first trimester of pregnancy, as it may bring on menses.

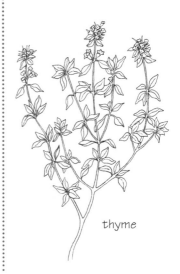

thyme

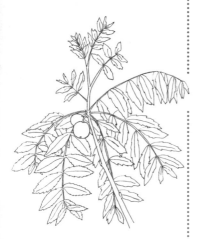

violet

walnut

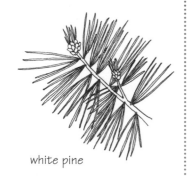

white pine

VIOLET (*VIOLA TRICOLOR, V. ODORATA, AND V. SPP.*)

The common Johnny-jump-up and heartsease (purple with heart-shaped leaves) are the two violas most commonly used medicinally. Drying destroys the pleasant aromas and flavors of violet, so use fresh. Syrups will preserve the flower for quite some time, however. Violet syrup will chase a cough away while pampering your taste buds. Fresh violet greens have a peppery taste that lifts otherwise dull salads and dishes. A high-end nutritive plant, violet is a common ingredient in most spring tonics.

WALNUT — BLACK WALNUT OR WHITE WALNUT (BUTTERNUT) (*JUGLANS NIGRA, J. CINEREA*)

Working with walnut is an exercise in patience and forethought. The husks, superb against parasites, fungal infection, and skin diseases, will leave your fingers stained brown for months. The nuts contain essential fatty acids, rebuild cellular strength, and are traditionally used to treat eczema internally. They are also notoriously difficult to crack. I use a vise and hammer, or roll over them with my car! Peeling the bark always frustrates me, but the bark is one of the few effective laxatives that is safe to use in pregnancy. Only the leaves are easy to gather, if you can reach them. But no matter: Walnut's reliability in treating these conditions makes it worth the effort. I admit I enjoy meeting the walnut's challenge.

WHITE PINE (*PINUS STROBUS* SPP.)

White pine is a first-aid station wrapped up in a tree. The sap makes an airtight, antiseptic, and pain-relieving bandage. I use it for all manner of burns, scrapes, and wounds. Cover with a tissue to stop the sap from sticking. Fishermen apply warm sap to stubborn splinters to draw them out painlessly. Some people have a skin sensitivity to pine sap — test it on a small patch of healthy skin for possible reaction before applying to a wide area.

The needles are a year-round source of vitamins C and A. They excel at breaking up congestion. Use as tea, steam pot, cough drops, or chest compress. The green bark makes a good splint for sprains, lending both support and pain relief.

Advantages of These Herbs

Obviously, there are many other herbs that can be used. But to start with, the twenty-five simples discussed in the previous section have several advantages. First, they are common through most of the United States, being easy to grow or readily available commercially. Second, wild populations of these plants are not threatened with overharvesting, as of this writing. Third, all are fairly easy to recognize in the field — with no extremely poisonous look-alikes. And, finally, all have flavors and scents appealing to most beginners.

CHOOSING THE HERB TO USE

The essence of herbal medicine is the quest for balance. Simply put, balance as a chronic state evokes health. Aristotle named it moderation and said "Man must enjoy his moderation, lest that, too, become excessive." At their best, medicinal plants become part of daily living, our food, thus preventing our tendency to swing from one extreme to another.

Seeking Balance

Some plants are balanced, or neutral in themselves, but most plants bring us away from excess because of the balancing work they can do for the body. Generally, I use a plant that has the opposite characteristics of the illness. Between the two (the illness and the herb), balance is found. For example, if the ailment is cold hands, use a plant that generates heat, such as ginger. If the cause of cold hands is poor circulation, look to an herb that promotes healthy circulation, such as strawberry, or to a nutritive herb such as viola to nourish overall health.

As the body moves toward balance, the herbal therapy needs of that body should be reevaluated. Perhaps the symptom of cold hands has disappeared. Is it because winter is over? Because circulation has improved? Each person must heed his own body's signals and rhythms to determine the next step. Perhaps the use of ginger can be discontinued. Perhaps the dose of nutritive herbs can be reduced to a maintenance level, or discontinued for a time to evaluate the results.

No matter what any herbal expert may tell you, you know your body best. Herbal healing is an art. There's no one best way — only the way that works best for the individual. Ultimately, you must find your own balance, or it really is not balance at all.

Working Inside and Out

A common method of herbal therapy is to treat the ailment internally and externally at the same time. To relieve severe colic or gas pain I might have the person rest with a warm poultice of catnip tea on his stomach, as well as drink frequent small sips of catnip tea.

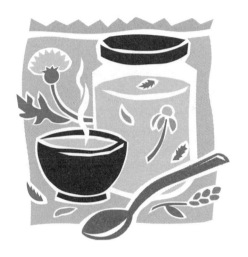

The Body of Herbalism: Preparing the Herbs

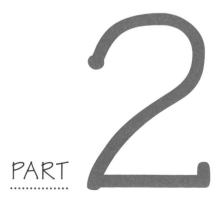

PART 2

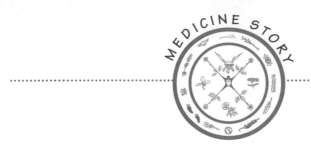

HOW WE GOT MEDICINE

When the world was young, the animals called a council. In those days, the beasts, birds, fishes, and insects could all understand each other. They and the people lived together in peace and friendship. But as time went on, the people increased so rapidly that they began to slaughter the larger creatures for their flesh or skin, while the smaller creatures were crushed.

Otter, the diplomat, led the council and soon the animals agreed to go to war with the people. But how? Then Coyote spoke up. "I can sneak into the people's village and find out what their weaknesses and strengths are." When he returned, he said, "What people have that we don't is a bow and arrow. If we had those tools, I know we could win."

Beaver remembered there was an old yew tree in a forest the people had burned down years ago. He went and cut it and shaped it into a bow. Reed said they could use her dried stalks for arrow shafts. Wild Turkey gave three of her best tail feathers. Flint dashed himself against some rocks under a waterfall to make a good arrowhead. The bow and arrow were all ready.

"Hold on . . . something's missing," said Snail, looking over the bow and arrow thoroughly. "This won't work." Then Coyote remembered about the bow string . . . he had seen the people twirl animal intestines to make the string. Well, you can imagine no one wanted to give up his intestines to make a string!

Then Old Cat stepped forward. She said, "I have no teeth and can't hunt any-more. I haven't eaten for a long time, and I'm tired. You can use my gut to help make the bow. I want to help, and it's really all I can do." Then she lay down and died. The animals thanked her for her gift. Her intestines made a strong and taut bowstring. But no one could pull the string.

You see, all the animals walked on four legs, or six, or had wings. Suddenly Bear drew himself upright. "See, I can stand like man. Give me time to practice, I'll work the bow." A week went by and Bear returned to the council. He said, "The bow works fine, but my claws keep getting in the way. I know if we could just cut them off somehow, then I could aim the arrow and kill the people."

"No, Bear!" Otter said. "If we cut off your claws, then you're no longer Bear. You can't climb a tree, fish, or grub for insects. You'll be no better than the people." And with that the council gave up, and was about to disband, when a small voice came out of the air.

"Ho! We can help. We can kill all the people!"

"Who are you? Where are you?"

"Oh, you can't see us. We are the invisible ones. We are disease. And we surely can kill all of the people. But first everyone must agree."

One by one all the beasts, all the fliers, the crawlers, the swimmers, the divers, all agreed to let disease kill the people. But when the plants were asked, they paused: "Wait. We've never really paid much attention to people. Let us watch them for a whole cycle of seasons. Come back in a year. Then we'll give you our answer."

A year passed. The council was called and the plants said, "Wait. We have watched the people, and you know, in a year's time, their babies can't speak for themselves yet. Come back in twenty years when they have grown to adults. Then we'll give you our answer."

Twenty years passed. The council was called and the plants said, "Wait. We have watched the people, and you know, in twenty years' time their hearts are still young. Come back in a hundred years when they have lived a whole lifetime. Then we'll give you our answer." The animals grumbled. A hundred years from now, would there even be any animals left? But they had no choice.

A hundred years passed. The council was called and the animals said, "No more delays. You must give your answer now, plants. Do we let disease go to war with the people or not?"

"Yes, go ahead," said the plants. "Do your worst. Give the people disease. You are right — the people destroy too much. We won't stop you."

"But," said the plants, "we did notice some people who are not like the rest. They show respect. They ask first, and they are careful. So we will help them. Anytime a person comes and asks us for help in a proper way, we will help."

And that is how we got medicine.

This story belongs to the Cherokee people. It was first recorded by James Mooney in 1890 in The Sacred Formulas of the Cherokees. I first heard it told by David Winston, a Cherokee herbal healer.

CHAPTER 4

Potent Potables: Making Herbal Tinctures

Alcohol is a good preservative for everything but brains.
— Mary Pettibone Poole, *A Glass Eye at the Keyhole*

Tinctures are simple and fun to make. Basically, the process of making a tincture involves extracting the virtues of the plant into an alcohol solution, simultaneously making and preserving the medicine. A mindfully made and stored tincture will generally be potent for about five years. Tinctures are convenient where time constraints or bitter tastes hinder the use of a tea. People often use tinctures for pets, for children, when traveling, or when bedridden.

The money you save from making your own tinctures is almost as good as having a winning lottery ticket. One day, I grabbed my shovel, set my stopwatch, and timed how long it took to make a dandelion root tincture. From digging to clean-up, making 1 quart of tincture took a grand total of 15 minutes of my time. The only cash expense was twelve dollars for the alcohol.

WHAT IS A "STANDARD DOSE" OF TINCTURE?

Different herbalists may suggest slightly different dosages for various tinctures, but one standard dosage for simple herbs that many follow is:

1 to 2 drops of 20 percent alcohol herb tincture for every 5 pounds of body weight, placed in an 8-ounce cup of water.

If I was buying that same dandelion root tincture, it would have cost me $4 per ounce on the average — that's $128 per quart! Subtract the $12 spent for the alcohol and I'm still left with a savings of $116 for 15 minutes' work, or $464 per hour!

CALCULATING STANDARD DOSAGE

Tinctures made from the simples recommended in this book are potent medicine. The dose of a tincture is measured in drops. A standard dose many herbalists follow is 1 to 2 drops of tincture for every 5 pounds of body weight, placed in an 8-ounce cup of water. For a baby less than six months old (who's suffering from colic, for example), the mother should take the tincture; the baby will receive the medicine through the mother's milk. For strong-tasting tinctures, disguise the drops in juice or food, or take them sublingually (under the tongue).

Frequency of Use

The frequency and duration of tincture use will vary depending on the illness. For acute conditions such as colds or earaches, take smaller doses more frequently, sometimes as often as ten times a day, with water. For nourishing the overall health or for treating chronic long-term conditions (such as recurring ear infections), take the standard dose two to four times a day for six to eight weeks, or longer if needed.

If an individual is sensitive to alcohol, simply place the drops of tincture into water that is just under the boiling point and let it sit for 5 minutes before drinking. The heat will evaporate most of the alcohol.

HOW TO MAKE A TINCTURE

Making a tincture as described on pages 50–52, with approximately equal amounts of 80-proof alcohol and plant material, yields a product that is roughly 20 percent alcohol. Anything from 15 percent to 25 percent alcohol will store nicely. Use a greater concentration of alcohol and you are not maximizing the herb's potential; use a lesser, and the tincture may mold or turn in storage. Makes about 12 ounces of finished tincture.

Materials
- ◆ Pint-size glass jar with tight-fitting lid
- ◆ About 2 cups fresh plant material of your choice (should fill jar leaving one inch of headroom)
- ◆ 2 cups 80-proof vodka, brandy, or rum

step 1

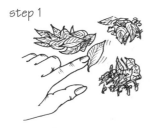

1. Clean and sort through your freshly gathered plants. Discard any yellow, moldy, damaged, or rotten parts. Separate out the parts you will be tincturing — flowers, leaves, or other parts. Wash off muddy roots. You may chop the herbs to help open the cell walls to the alcohol. This speeds up the process, which is useful if you want to start using the tincture in one to two weeks.

step 2

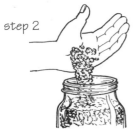

2. Fill the glass jar with the plant material, leaving about 1 inch for headroom.

step 3

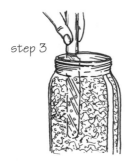

3. Completely cover the herb with vodka, brandy, or rum. Insert a butter knife into the jar and run it around the inside the jar to release any trapped air bubbles. Add more alcohol to cover. Put on the lid and shake vigorously for about 1 minute.

step 4

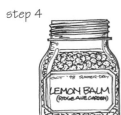

4. Label and date each tincture. If you have room on the label, note what the weather and seasonal conditions were when you gathered the herbs. This will help you identify and track the best gathering times for various herbs (see box).

step 5

5. Place the jar in a dark place and let it sit for 3 to 6 weeks. Shake periodically, and check to make sure that the plant material remains covered with alcohol. Add alcohol as needed.

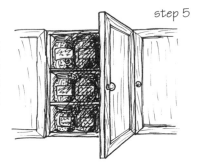

6. After 3 to 6 weeks have passed and the plant material looks pale, limp, and spent, strain and press the liquid through a piece of cheesecloth into a glass or stainless steel bowl or pitcher, leaving the plant material behind in the jar or on the cheesecloth.

step 6

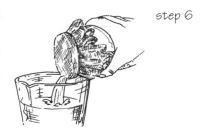

7. Once you've poured out all the liquid, spoon out all the herbs onto the cheesecloth. Wrap the cheesecloth around the herbs, hold over the bowl or pitcher, and wring out any additional tincture.

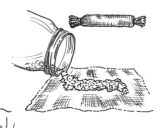

step 7

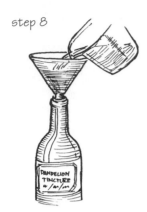

step 8

8. Using a funnel, if desired, pour the tincture into a glass bottle of the appropriate size. Label, date, and store the bottle in a cool dark place.

Now, to be honest, I don't always get to the last three steps right away. I have jars of tinctures several years old sitting on my shelves that still have not been strained. The alcohol keeps the plant preserved. I rather enjoy looking at the preserved plants, and just strain some tincture off to use as needed.

Variations on Method

Using stronger-proof alcohol. If you use 190-proof alcohol to make a tincture, remember you are now working with alcohol that has only 5 percent water. You will have to add some water so the water-soluble components of the herb can be extracted, or use extra amounts of fresh plant material, which contain their own water. The proportion can be increased to one part alcohol to 4 or 5 parts fresh plant material. A simple way to do this is to run the tincture through two or three times.

Thus for a red clover tincture, I'll gather plant material and prepare the tincture once. Two to 3 weeks later, I'll strain and repack the fluid with yet another picking of red clover. This obviously makes a stronger medicine, so the dosage should be less — roughly 1 to 2 drops per every 10 pounds of body weight. This is a bit more work, but some plants such as ginger, burdock, and poplar buds need the higher concentration of 190-proof alcohol to extract their resins and essential oils.

Juicing the herb. If you happen to have a juicer, you can press the juice from the fresh herb and mix that with an equal amount of 80-proof alcohol to yield a 20 percent alcohol tincture. (One and one-half parts juice to 1 part alcohol will yield a 16 percent alcohol tincture.) Alternatively, you can blend 1 part 190-proof alcohol with 4 parts juice to yield a 19 percent alcohol tincture. (Five parts juice to 1 part alcohol will yield a 15 percent alcohol tincture.)

Using dried herbs. Although fresh plant tinctures are usually preferable, dried plant tinctures are an acceptable alternative. Here are the steps to follow:

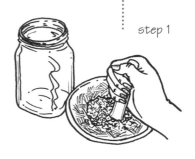

step 1

1. Grind 4 ounces of the dried herb to a powder using a mortar and pestle.

2. Place the herbs into a 1-pint glass jar.

3. Fill the jar to the top with 80-proof alcohol. Shake vigorously every day. From this point, follow the instructions for fresh herb tinctures (see step 4, page 50), but let the herbs settle before decanting the liquid into the glass jar for storage.

Glycerates Instead of Alcohol

For alcohol-sensitive individuals or for children, consider making a glycerate instead of an alcohol-based tincture. Glycerin is a thick, sweet, and slippery-feeling liquid. It helps mask the taste of bitter herbs such as dandelion, so children like it better. It extracts most plant alkaloids and mucilages (the slippery quality of mallow root), but will not extract resins (found in poplar, white pine, and ginger). Follow the guidelines for the standard tincture dose on page 49, substituting the glycerin for alcohol guidelines.

Making a glycerate. For a fresh-herb glycerate, follow the steps on pages 50–52, substituting equal amounts of 100-percent vegetable glycerin and distilled water for the 80-proof alcohol. (Since 80-proof alcohol comes already diluted with water, we must dilute the 100-percent glycerin with water to get a similar dilution.)

You'll find some herbalists prefer a two-to-one ratio of glycerin to water, since fresh herbs already bring their own natural water to the tincture. So there is some room for experimentation

ONE HERB AT A TIME

Make your tincture only with a single herb at first. Once you have a variety of single-herb tinctures, you can combine them in different proportions as needed. When you find a particularly useful or favorite combination, then consider making the blend from a combination of fresh herbs.

on our part. Do try to keep the final glycerin ratio to at least 25 percent to reduce the risk of spoilage and for safe consumption, since excessive amounts of glycerates may cause diarrhea in sensitive individuals.

To make a glycerate with dried herbs, remember to add extra distilled water to replace the water that has been evaporated out. A proportion of 4 ounces of dried herb, 1½ cups of distilled water, and ½ cup of vegetable glycerin will yield you a 25 percent glycerate. Follow the steps for making dried herb tinctures listed on page 53.

TINCTURE BLEND RECIPES

The following recipes are some of my family's and students' favorites. These represent a variety of blends that are useful to have on hand and ready to use. Once you've tried making some of these, you may want to create your own blends, or adapt these recipes. See chapter 9 for guidance in how to develop blends.

Making Blended Tinctures

You will notice that some of these recipes call for gathering flowers in the spring and roots in the fall. Follow the same procedure for making fresh herb tinctures on pages 50–52, only turn it into a two step process: First, tincture your fresh gathered spring flowers and allow the tincture to sit unstrained until you gather your fresh root in the fall. Just remove the spent

---

A NOTE ON MEASURING

The proportions of herbs in these recipes are referred to as parts. How much a part is, is up to you — it could be a gram, an ounce, a pound, depending on how much tincture you want to make and how much plant material you have available. The important thing is that the relative amounts, or parts, are followed closely. It is always more precise to measure by weight, and it's important that you use the same method of measurement for all the ingredients in a particular recipe.

flowers from the tincture, wringing out as much liquid as possible. then use this flower tincture as the base. Now add your roots and begin the tincturing process a second time.

DIGESTIVE BITTERS

This blend stimulates appetite, aids digestion, and reduces nausea. Pregnant women looking to ease morning sickness should leave out the ginger. Instead add a little ginger as a food flavoring. It will still help suppress nausea. Current guidelines state that while ginger is safe for pregnant women when used as a food, it should be used in moderation as a medicine as it may stimulate uterine activity in the early stages of pregnancy. It's also nice for colic, or colds and flus that affect the digestive system. For extreme nausea, take only 1 teaspoon of the standard dose diluted in a cup of water (see page 48), every ten minutes; most of the time this small amount can be kept down. This also makes a nice blend to add to an herbal wine or syrup.

> 1 part catnip bud or leaf (calms nervous stomach)
> 1 part grated gingerroot (dispels indigestion, flatulence, and nausea)
> 1 part fall-gathered dandelion root (aids in the absorption of food)
> 1 part mallow root (soothes the digestive tract)

REJUVENATING FEMALE TONIC

This tonic helps maintain and build the body's strength before and after pregnancy, during nursing, through menopause, and after a miscarriage or abortion; it also eases chronic menstrual cramping.

> ½ part borage leaf (maintains adrenal health)
> ½ part lemon balm leaf (lifts spirits)
> 2 parts fresh raspberry leaf (strengthens female reproductive system)
> 1 part violet blossom and leaf (tonic to whole system)
> 1 part burdock root (promotes liver function)
> 1 part plantain leaf (nourishing and soothing to internal membranes)

COLD SEASON REMEDY

This tastes like medicine — though pleasantly so. I like to take it sweetened with honey and a couple of wedges of fresh lemon. As soon as everyone else around me is getting sick, I start dosing myself with this formula, along with taking a clove or two of garlic. This is the one tincture I always try to have on hand, because when the whole household is sick, I don't always have the time or energy to keep brewing tea.

½ part inner poplar bark (anti-inflammatory and
   pain relieving)
½ part mullein leaf (helps prevent cold from settling
   into lungs)
1 part thyme leaf (antiviral and antibiotic)
1 part lemon balm leaf (lifts spirits)
1 part mallow root (soothes inflamed tissues and serves as
   expectorant)
1 part violet leaf and flower (soothes inflamed tissues and
   serves as expectorant)
1 part peppermint leaf (reduces nausea and fever, works
   as stimulant)

DIARRHEA OR DYSENTERY BLEND

This is another good tincture to have on hand ready to use at a moment's notice. Diarrhea can come on quickly and severely and there is danger of dehydration. This formula helps stop the runs and prevent the electrolyte imbalance that can result from severe dehydration.

To administer, take small frequent sips of the standard dose with a tablespoon of vinegar added to it.

2 parts blackberry root (astringent)
1 part alfalfa leaf (helps replace lost minerals)
1 part mallow root (soothes irritated tissues)
1 part red rose petal (astringent)

LESS STRESS BLEND

This blend helps build the body's capacity to cope with stress while simultaneously calming the nervous system and easing depression. Besides taking this formula, rich in oat straw, try to eat lots of foods containing oats, which nourish the nervous system.

1 part fresh young strawberry leaf (considered a centering herb; see page 146. It's also a rich source of vitamins, especially vitamin C.)
1 part lemon balm leaf (uplifts spirits)
2 parts St.-John's-wort blossom (combats depression)
1 part lavender blossom (combats nervous exhaustion)
2 parts green oat straw (nourishes the nervous system)
¼ part crushed borage seeds (maintains adrenal health)
¼ part crushed plantain seeds (high in B vitamins and soothes irritated tissues)

SKIN WASH

For external use only, this tincture could be made with less expensive rubbing or isopropyl alcohol, or with vinegar. Dilute to the standard dose with water and use a topical application for all manner of skin parasites, fungi, poison ivy rashes, impetigo, or other irritated, wet, itchy skin conditions.

2 parts black or white walnut leaf (antifungal and antiseptic)
1 part rose leaf (astringent)
1 part St.-John's-wort blossom (promotes rapid healing)
1 part thyme leaf (antiseptic)

MAKE YOUR OWN NATURAL PRESERVATIVE

A tincture made from the buds of the balsam poplar acts as a natural preservative. A few drops of this tincture added to oils, syrups, wines, and vinegars you make (see recipes in following chapters) will keep these formulas from turning and give them a longer shelf life.

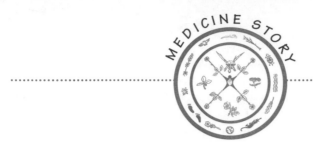
THE GREAT TREE

When the world was young, there was one huge tree that bore all kinds of delicious fruits, nuts, and vegetables. Plump ears of corn, huge plums, stalks of wild rice, large hazelnuts all hung from its branches. If you were hungry, you could just pick a leaf from the tree and sweet maple syrup would stream out from its stalk. All the people depended on this tree for their food.

Nanaboozhoo came walking by one day to get a bit of fruit to eat for himself. At the foot of the tree, the people were standing about, stuffing themselves as fast as they could. Nanaboozhoo tried to get closer, but the people crowded him out of the way. The more he tried, the more the people pushed him away.

Finally, Nanaboozhoo became so angry he tore the tree out of the ground, smashed it into pieces, and left. The people grew sad at the loss of this giant tree, and when winter came, they were hungry. They asked Nanaboozhoo for help. Now, Nanaboozhoo didn't want to be mean, it was just that sometimes he couldn't help himself. So he said, "When the snows melt, plant the branches and plant the leaves." That spring, wherever the people put a branch or a leaf into the ground, a different fruit or vegetable grew. All the food grew as separate plants, and had to be cultivated by the people from then on.

The trunk of the great tree grew to be beautiful sugar maple. When a leaf was picked, thick syrup still streamed forth. Pretty soon, the people lay all day drinking the maple syrup, and when Nanaboozhoo went to have some, it was all gone. So he stood over the maple and urinated gallons and gallons right into the tree until the syrup flowed like water. Ever since, maple sap has to be boiled down to make syrup. Wood has to be cut, fires must be kept up, everyone has to work together, and the trees have to be tended. The people are too busy to bother Nanaboozhoo much anymore.

In the northern woodlands, the trees and forests are what cathedrals are to Europe. There is the Great Tree of Life, the Great Tree of Peace, and here we have all cultivated food springing from another Great Tree. I first heard a version of this story at a Three Fires gathering from a Canadian Chippewa-Cree woman. It's also partly recorded in Chief Andrew Blackbird's accounts of Nanaboozhoo's deeds.

CHAPTER 5

Practical Pampering:
Making Herb Oils and Salves

▼▼▼

But let us hence, my sovereign, to provide
a salve for any sore that may betide

— William Shakespeare, *Henry III*

Every single day someone in our household reaches for a jar of herb oil or salve. With a family of six, I make herb oils in large batches and store them in the refrigerator so they last as long as possible. With an herb oil in hand, turning it into a salve, ointment, sachet, or balm (all are different terms for essentially the same product) is simply a matter of adding a thickening agent, beeswax being the easiest and most commonly used. Once the word gets out that you make your own oils and salves, expect to make some for friends and relatives. Show them how to use it, and be sure they actually want the product before you give it away: It is heartbreaking to see a jar of your precious home-made salve just sitting on a shelf for years.

HOW TO MAKE AN INFUSED-HERB OIL

When you begin experimenting with this process, I recommend making a basic herb oil with a single herb. Just as with tinctures, most people prefer to make up several different oils and then blend them together when needed to create a blended oil. Sometimes, though, you will have a specific use for an oil or salve in mind and will want to make a blended-herb oil. Following are the steps for making a single-herb oil for external use. The amounts given will make about 5 ounces of herb oil, but you do not need to follow these proportions exactly. How much herb oil you make depends on how much of the herb you have and the desired strength of the finished oil. The basic principle is simply to cover the herbs with oil and allow them to steep.

If you use the preservation techniques I recommend in step 3, the oil should have a shelf life of six months to one year when stored in the refrigerator. Makes about 5 ounces of herb oil.

Materials
- ½ pint widemouthed mason jar with 2-part lid
- About ¾ cup herb of your choice
- ¾ cup oil of your choice (see page 62)
- About 2 tablespoons 190-proof alcohol
- A few drops of balsam poplar tincture (optional) (see page 38)

1. Gather the fresh herbs of your choice. Shake the dirt off the leaves or wash and blot dry the roots. Sort out and discard any diseased plant material. Make a pile of the part of the herb you wish to use. Chop it coarsely until you have about ¾ cup.

2. Mold and fungus grow easily in oils, so allow the herb to partially wilt overnight to reduce moisture content. The volume of the herb will also reduce.

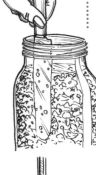

3. Fill a glass jar with the herbs. Leave about 2 inches of headroom. Cover the herb with oil. Insert a butter knife into the jar and run it along the inside of the jar to eliminate any trapped air bubbles. Make sure the oil covers the herbs completely: you may need to add a little more oil.

I like to float a ½-inch layer of 190-proof alcohol on top (vodka would work also). The alcohol helps prevent airborne molds from turning your oil and helps draw the plant essences into the oil. I also add a couple of drops of balsam poplar tincture on top as a natural preservative. Cover with tight fitting lid and shake vigorously for about a minute. Remove the lid.

4. Cover the jar with four layers of cheesecloth, secure with the outer ring of the jar lid or a rubber band, and place it in a warm dry spot (such as a sunny windowsill or on top of a water heater) for about 2 weeks, or until the oil has taken on the color of the herbs and the alcohol has evaporated. I have also had success setting the herbs in a slow-cooker on a low setting or in a yogurt maker for several days. Some people prefer to simmer their herbs on the stove for a couple of hours. While this does make the oil quickly, I find its end product generally pales in comparison to those of the slower methods.

5. Finally, strain the oil through cheesecloth or mesh strainer into a bowl, pressing out as much oil from the herbs as possible. Let the oil sit overnight. Decant the oil to separate it from any sediment or water that may have settled to the bottom. To decant, simply pour the top oil off slowly. As the bottom sediment comes to the edge, stop pouring. Let settle. You can use a turkey baster to siphon off the remaining oil resting on top of the sediment. Store the oil in a capped glass jar in the refrigerator or another cool dark place until needed. Label and date the oil.

HOW TO MAKE A SALVE FROM AN HERB OIL

When kept in the refrigerator, salves seem to have a longer shelf life than herb oils — often twice as long, or up to two years.

Materials
- ◆ Double boiler
- ◆ 1 tablespoon (15 ml) beeswax
- ◆ Other nutrients, as desired

step 1

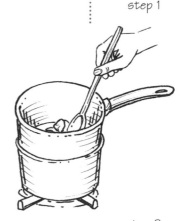

1. Gently warm 8 liquid ounces of herb oil in a glass or stainless-steel double boiler. Add 1 tablespoon of beeswax. Experiment with adding small amounts (about ½ teaspoon at a time) of other enriching ingredients, such as lanolin, vitamin E oil, cocoa butter, coconut oil, balsam poplar bud oil, or balsam poplar bud tincture. Add only a few drops of the tincture at a time, or separation may occur.

step 2

2. When the ingredients are melted together, check the consistency by placing a drop or two of the salve in ice water. If the salve is thick, it will form into a little ball. If it's thinner, the oil will spread out over the surface. Add small amounts of beeswax (¼ teaspoon at a time) to firm the salve, or slightly larger amounts of herb oil (one teaspoon at a time) to thin the salve.

3. While the mixture is still liquid, pour it into a shallow large-mouthed glass jar, or a container you can easily get your fingers into to reach the salve. Let sit until cool. If salve is not of your desired firmness, place the jar into a hot water bath until the salve is again liquid. Play with adjusting the proportions of oil to beeswax until you are happy with your results. Keep notes; you'll appreciate it for the next batch! Label and date the jar. To store a salve for future use, pour melted beeswax on the top to seal it from decay.

Add a touch of whimsy to your home-made salves by using unusual containers. For example, seashells or a hollowed-out birch log make practical nonreactive containers, and unique gifts.

RECIPES FOR OILS AND SALVES

Using these basic techniques, you can make your oils and salves with single herbs or in combinations. If you have a sense of what you will be using the salve for before you start making it, then you can select the most appropriate herbs and proportions for each to treat a particular ailment. Have some fun experimenting to develop your own oil combinations, and discovering your personal favorites. Following are a few of my own favorites.

HOW THICK DO YOU WANT YOUR SALVE?

The consistency, or thickness, of your salve can be varied by the amount of herb oil to beeswax you use. Your choice will depend on how you intend to use the salve. A thicker, waxier salve is best for rubbing into cracks around knuckle joints, or for lip balms and sachets. A softer, oilier salve is preferable for massage oils and liniments, where it will be applied over a larger area of the body.

HUNTER'S HAND AND FOOT RUB

This is a favorite salve for bringing heat to an area and providing a measure of pain relief. Rub on your chest and sinuses to break up congestion, on your feet at the end of a long day, on your hands before going out to work in cold soil, or on sore muscles. It can also be used as a daily application to get rid of those tiny red spider veins that form on legs, arms, neck, and face. *Warning:* Don't use this salve near your eyes or delicate tissues. Use 190-proof alcohol when making this herb oil to be sure to extract the essences of ginger and poplar into the oil.

- 1 part inner poplar bark (reduces inflammation and relieves pain)
- 1 part grated fresh gingerroot (increases circulation)

NOT FOR WOMEN ONLY

This blend has a spicy clean scent that appeals to both men and women. Use it as a massage oil or thicken it to make a salve to soothe chapped lips or mild sunburn. My daughter likes to dab a little of the salve behind her ears as a perfume sachet — so does her father, and I like the scent when he does!

- 1 part lavender blossom (spicy scent, topically healing, and antiseptic)
- 1 part wild rose petal (soothing scent, astringent, and anti-inflammatory)

CAUTION ON OILS

Never use essential oils in place of homemade infused oils: They are *not* interchangeable. Essential oils are the concentrated distilled essences of plants; it may take as much as a pound of lavender to make a few drops of essential oil. They are nearly always diluted before use and seldom applied directly onto the skin or used internally. All the recipes for oils in this book incorporate only infused oils. Do not use essential oils in their place unless appropriate reductions in measurements are made and the oils are properly diluted!

ALL-PURPOSE SALVE

This multipurpose salve provides relief to sore muscles, reduces inflammation, heals scrapes, relieves minor burns, and even provides a measure of protection from biting insects. Excellent chest rub to break up congestion.

1 part plantain leaf (topically healing and soothing)
1 part lavender blossom (antiseptic, topically healing, pain relieving, repels insects)
1 part peppermint leaf (cooling, antispasmodic, and pain relieving)
1 part thyme leaf (antiseptic and antifungal, increases blood flow to the area, healing and astringent)

GENTLE SALVE

This blend is suitable for all manner of sore or chapped skin that accompanies having babies, including cracked nipples, chapped bottoms, perineal stitches, stretch marks, and diaper rash. It can also be used safely on delicate elderly skin. It relieves inflammation, is mildly antimicrobial, and soothes irritated tissues.

2 parts plantain leaf (topically healing)
1 part violet flowers (soothing, healing, and antimicrobial in action)
1 part mullein flowers (reduces swelling and inflammation)

FAST-HEALING SALVE

This salve promotes rapid cell growth so wounds heal quickly with reduced scarring. Do not to use this salve over infected or dirty skin, as new tissue can grow right over the infection, complicating the wound.

2 parts St.-John's-wort flower (stimulates nerve endings to heal)
1 part balsam poplar buds (antiinflammatory, antiseptic, and paints a thin protective resin over cut to keep wound clean)
1 part crushed rose hips (or vitamin E oil: 1 tablespoon vitamin E oil to every 4 tablespoons herb oil)

Optional ingredient: 1 part white pine pitch, for a salve effective against those cracks you get in the sides of your fingers from working in the garden too much (chilblains)

ANTIFUNGAL SALVE

These herbs may be made into a salve, to help heal broken and cracked skin, or a vinegar (see page 76), to help relieve itching when the skin is not broken. Dilute vinegar by two-thirds with water before applying to cracked or open tissues. It stains the skin, as iodine does. This formula works well for athlete's foot, ringworm, and ectopic or eczematous skin conditions.

> 1 part walnut husks (antifungal)
> 1 part thyme leaf (antiseptic)
> 1 part rose leaf (astringent)
> 1 part plantain leaf (soothing)

BORAGE OIL

The seeds from borage (and evening primrose) contain a special substance called gamma linoleic acid, also known as GLA. GLA (naturally occurring in human breast milk) helps correct metabolic imbalances in the body and inflammations that stem from a degeneration of organic processes. It is most often used to help restore balance during recovery from alcoholism, during weight loss, to ease premenstrual syndrome and arthritis, soothe infantile eczema, and reduce irritable bowel syndrome; it's also a quick remedy for hangovers. Both borage oil and evening primrose oil are readily available at most health food stores — be sure it has been cold expressed and not chemically extracted. The oil should be taken internally several times daily and, for quicker relief, be simultaneously applied externally to the affected regions.

GATHERING MULLEIN

I enjoy picking mullein flowers — it is an exercise in patience that takes me past the work and becomes a form of movement meditation. But if I have a busy schedule which limits the time I can spend picking, then the slow pace becomes frustrating instead of calming. A shortcut is to gather the entire flower spike and chop it up finely. One flower spike is generally enough to fulfill my family's needs for the year. Gather the spike just above the last set of leaves to allow the mullein plant to grow another spike.

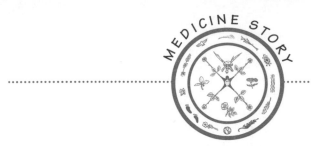

HOW WE GOT MAPLE SYRUP

Once, a beautiful young maiden was taken captive by a warring tribe. She soon realized the journey back to her people was too difficult to manage on her own, so she made up her mind to learn the ways of her captors. Now, her captors were harsh to her at first, but after she learned their language she was no longer treated as a captive, and she was called Moqua.

A young warrior became fond of Moqua and they married. At first, Moqua worked hard to always have a warm fire and good food waiting for her husband when he returned from hunting. But as her skill grew at her tasks she found she could have everything done by midmorning. Then she'd spend the rest of the day visiting with friends. One spring day she was in such a hurry to go visiting, she didn't want to waste time gathering the cooking water.

So instead of getting water to add to the meat pot, Moqua quickly poured the maple sap her husband saved for his evening drink into the pot, thinking, "I'll gather more sap later to replace it — he'll never notice." She put on a big chunk of beechwood so the fire would last a very long time, set the meat pot off to the side to slowly simmer, then left for the rest of the day.

Moqua had such a good time that she didn't notice it was getting dark. She hurried home, worried her husband would be angry that she hadn't replaced the maple sap she'd taken. When she returned, he sat waiting for her, but a grin was on his face. "What did you do to this meat?" he asked. "It is the best I've ever had. Why, I want you to cook it like this every time!"

Puzzled, Moqua peered into the kettle. She saw that the meat was sticky, and it tasted sweet and wonderful. She noticed little grains of something like sand at the bottom and wondered if, perhaps, the maple sap had made this? So she washed her kettle, then poured in the last bit of the maple sap. She set it on the fire to boil. Then she set it outside in the snow to cool. The result was maple sugar. The fame of Moqua's skill in cooking soon spread everywhere. And Moqua's husband always helped her gather and cook the sap every spring to be sure of his wonderful dinners.

Versions of this story are common throughout maple sugar country. Most of this area shares a common linguistic root — the Algonquian. Though each tribe may claim to have been the first to make maple syrup, the ultimate credit goes to Moqua, the captive who made many mistakes.

CHAPTER 6
Homespun Alchemy: Making Medicinal Wines and Vinegars

▼▼▼▼▼

"Just living is not enough," said the butterfly.
"One must have sunshine, freedom, and a little flower."
— Hans Christian Andersen

Winemaking has been around far longer than the specialty homebrewing supply shops that sell all kinds of paraphernalia, from fermentation locks to expensive and delicate yeasts, cadmium tablets, and even glass bottles and corks! Being a tightwad at heart, I wondered just how *did* they used to make wine without all that fancy equipment, and could I replicate the process in my own home?

I headed over to my local library to research an old English and Celtic form of wine called mead. What I found out was that not only were wines once made from fruit, but herbs were added as well, to give unique flavors, scents, and healing properties. I have been hooked on winemaking ever since.

Making wine relies on the slow process of fermentation for preservation. Fermentation happens naturally as plants are left exposed to air and rot. While they do so, airborne yeasts and bacteria break down sugar and starch. Alcohol is excreted in the process. The yeasts and bacteria keep producing alcohol, until eventually the environment becomes toxic to them and they die. This is what forms the sediment in your bottles of homemade wine and vinegar. The trick is to control this process to yield a desirable product.

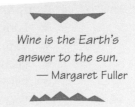

Wine is the Earth's answer to the sun.
— Margaret Fuller

HOW TO MAKE MEDICINAL HERB WINE

It usually takes about 2 months to make a batch of wine from start to finish, but I actually put in only about 2 to 3 hours' effort in all. Fermentation can be smelled by every wild animal living in your county — they also consider wine a delicacy — so find a critter-safe area for your fermenting brew.

When starting out, you will probably want to produce several small experimental batches. Once you have your recipe down, you'll find it is more economical to make larger batches. With experience, you're also likely to want to give the finished wine a longer time to age and mellow. Following are proportions for both small and large batches. Note that the proportions are slightly different for the larger batch.

For small experimental batches:

Yield: about 1 gallon without sediment

1–2	quarts (1–2 liters) fruit (optional)
1½	gallons (6 liters) water
1	pound (400 g) honey (or other sugar source)
1	tablespoon (15 ml) baker's yeast
½–1	pound (200–400 g) herbs
1	pound (400 g) dried fruit

For larger batches:

Yield: About 4 gallons without sediment

4	quarts (4 liters) fruit (optional)
5	gallons (19 liters) water
3	pounds (1 kilogram) honey
1	tablespoon (15 ml) baker's yeast
3–5	pounds (1–2.25 kilograms) herbs
3	pounds (1 kilogram) dried fruit

Equipment:

- ◆ Long-handled stirring spoon
- ◆ Paring knife
- ◆ Masher or grinder, to prepare fruit and herbs (optional)
- ◆ Large crock pot or other container made of glass or stainless steel; or an oak barrel (I've even used a 5-gallon plastic bucket — not my first choice, but better than not making wine at all)
- ◆ Three to four 750 ml bottles for each gallon of wine
- ◆ Containers for siphoning
- ◆ Cheesecloth
- ◆ Rubber bands
- ◆ Plastic tubing

1. Sterilize all the equipment you will use, including the containers for siphoning, with peroxide (see pages 23–24) or by boiling for 10 minutes.

2. Gather your fruits and herbs of choice. Clean them, sorting out and disposing of any debris or moldy- or diseased-looking pieces. Mash or cut the fresh (not the dried) fruit into 1-inch chunks. Cut any herb roots into 1-inch pieces or grind them coarsely. A food processor works well for this.

3. Place all the fruits and herbs into a large ceramic crock or other nonreactive container. (Although many herbalists like to decoct and strain the herbs first, I find that even hard roots such as burdock yield their virtues through fermentation. I simply strain and press out the herbs at the end.) Add the water, honey, and yeast, but make sure your container is only three-fourths full to allow room for expansion. Stir until well dissolved.

step 3

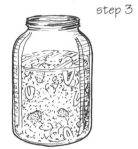

step 4

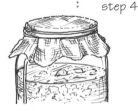

4. Cover with three layers of cheesecloth to allow the gases to exchange while preventing flies and renegade yeasts from getting in. Secure cheesecloth with a rubber band or string.

step 5

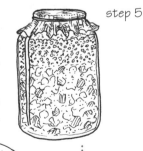

5. Set in a warm place (about 75˚–90˚F). Soon you will see bubbles start to rise. This is the start of fermentation, and means everything is working fine. After 5 to 7 days you'll notice the fermentation process noticeably slowing down (the bubbling is less active but not altogether gone).

step 6

6. Add the dried fruit. Cover with clean cheesecloth. Let sit undisturbed until all fermentation (bubbling) stops — about 3 to 6 weeks, depending on the temperature.

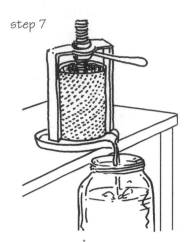

step 7

7. Strain all plant material out of the wine, using a press, a rice strainer, or a food mill to extract as much liquid from the plant material as possible. If you do not have any of this equipment, strain the wine through clean cheesecloth, then wrap the herbs in the cheesecloth and wring out the additional liquid; in larger batches, you may get as much as an additional gallon from this squeezing. Let the wine sit undisturbed in the original container or another large nonreactive container covered with clean cheesecloth for 24 hours to settle.

8. You will notice a layer of sediment on the bottom. Either decant the clear liquid slowly and then use a turkey baster to get the last bit out, or set up a simple siphon.

To make a siphon you need two equal-size containers and about 3 feet of ½-inch plastic tubing. Place the container holding the wine on a table, and place the other empty container on the floor. Fill the tube completely with water, pinching both ends to seal it. Hold one end over a sink or extra container at a lower level. Place the other end in the container holding the wine, and then release the tube, allowing the water to flow out until the tube is filled with wine. Then pinch the end of the tube. Transfer that end into the empty container on the floor, and allow gravity to do its work. Monitor the siphon in the wine to make sure it does not get down into the sediment and start siphoning off that as well.

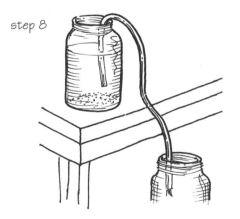

step 8

Use a simple siphon to draw the clear liquid from the higher container, leaving the sediment behind.

9. Pour the wine into sterilized wine bottles. I used to cork the bottles right away, but not anymore. If the fermentation isn't fully complete, the gas can pop the cork right out, leaving a big mess to clean up. To ensure complete fermentation, use a small deflated balloon as a test. Simply slip the balloon over the top of the bottle and watch for 24 hours. If there is any fermentation, escaping gas will inflate the balloon. Let the gas out of the balloon, and keep testing until the balloon remains deflated for 24 hours. Then cork, label, and date the bottles. You may cover the cork with melted beeswax to ensure a proper seal.

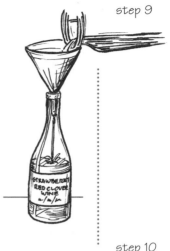

step 9

10. Store your wine in a cool dark place for at least 6 months. This allows for harsh flavors to blend and mellow. Keep corked bottles stored on their sides; otherwise the corks will dry out and there will no longer be a proper seal.

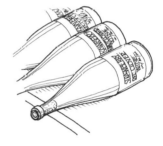

step 10

FAVORITE MEDICINAL WINE RECIPES

Winemaking fosters the creative impulse — have fun mulling over all the possible fruit and herb combinations before making a batch. If you can't decide whether to make lavender-strawberry wine or lavender–rose hip wine, a good way to sample potential flavor combinations is to first make a small pot of tea from the ingredients and do a taste test.

STANDARD DOSAGE FOR MEDICINAL WINE

The standard dose for medicinal wines is 1 to 2 ounces taken one to three times daily as needed. For children, I'll pour just-under-boiling water over the wine and let it rest for 5 minutes before serving. A little sweetener may be necessary.

I like to choose a fruit that has medicinal virtues suitable to the purpose of the wine. For example, for a wine designed to promote cardiac circulation, I would choose to use the circulation-enhancing fruit strawberry instead of raspberry or blackberry.

WINE TONIC FOR IMPROVED CIRCULATION

For fruit:
Fresh ripe strawberries

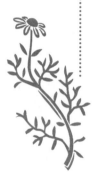

For herbs, combine:
2 parts red clover blossom (nourishing herb with mild blood-thinning properties)
1 part alfalfa leaf (provides trace minerals)
1 part lavender flower (eases depression and aids digestion)
½ part violet blossom (gentle circulatory stimulant)
½ part whole crushed rose hips (rich source of vitamin E)

REJUVENATING WINE TONIC

This formula is especially good for rebuilding strength from exhaustion, after pregnancy, from nursing, or after a long illness.

For fruit:
Raspberry, with 1 orange added per 1 gallon water

For herbs, combine:
1 part violet blossom and leaf (nourishing, diuretic, and anti-inflammatory)
2 parts borage leaf (maintains adrenal health)
1 part lemon balm leaf (uplifts spirits)
1 part green oat straw, with developing seed head (nourishes nervous system, soothing)
1 part alfalfa leaf (rejuvenating and nourishing)

GARLIC WINE

Make just enough of this wine for one day's use, since it should be used fresh; many of the active principles in the garlic will be lost by the next day.

1 fresh clove garlic, crushed
3 ounces (75 g) wine

Add the crushed garlic to the wine and let it rest for 10 to 15 minutes.

For external use: Apply this wine as a wash, or moisten a cloth and lay the garlic wine on as a dressing.
For internal use: Sip the 3-ounce glass of wine slowly throughout the day.

THE ORIGINS OF GARLIC WINE

The use of garlic wine dates back to the Greek physician Dioscorides, who administered it to the Roman Army. Dioscorides was also a famous Greek herbalist, responsible for devising the method of cataloging medicinal items still used by modern pharmacists.

His list of recommended applications for garlic wine is impressive: treating chronic coughs, healing wounds cleanly, preventing infections, dispelling toxic poisoning from bites of bees and scorpions, preventing and eliminating internal parasites, preventing food poisoning, clearing the arteries, preventing the spread of infectious diseases, and as a disinfectant wash. Garlic poultices were used for treating wartime injuries all the way up through World War I, when it was applied as a wound dressing, saving the limbs and lives of tens of thousands of soldiers.

Digestive Bitters

Bitters help balance overly sweet and salty diets. They activate digestive enzymes and bring warmth to the digestive process, helping the body break down and properly absorb the nutrients in our food. Most often they are used moderately in cooking or drunk just before eating.

BITTERS 1

For fruit:
Apples, or an equal amount of apples and oranges (quartered)

For herbs combine:
1 part fall-gathered dandelion root (promotes secretion of bile and helps with digestive absorption)
1 part mallow root (soothing)
1 part burdock root (aids liver function)
½ part thyme leaf (stimulates digestion)
½ lavender blossom (stimulates digestion)
½ part gingerroot — if you like a ginger "bite" and want a bitters that is aggressively warming (perhaps to balance a vegan diet), double the amount

BITTERS 2: DANDELION WINE

Dandelion wine makes an excellent digestive bitters all on its own. Take a 1-ounce serving of the wine fifteen to twenty minutes before eating. It can also be taken after a heavy meal to aid digestion.

For fruit:
1 lemon and 1 orange per 1 gallon (4 liters) of water

For herbs:
Dandelion flowers, picked early in the day

BITTERS 3

For children or those with sensitive, spasmodic stomachs.

For fruit:
Apples

For herbs, combine:
1 part catnip flower (calms nervous stomachs)
1 part dandelion flower (aids digestive process)
1 part mallow root (soothes irritated tissues)
1 part plantain leaf (soothes and heals)

Flower Wines

Basically any edible flower can be made into a wine. Some flowers are slightly insipid; adding a lemon will give their wines a little lift. You can also add a few walnut leaves for a drier, higher-tannin wine. One popular flower wine is, of course, rose petal, but lavender flower is equally sublime. A favorite of mine is blue wine made from borage, violet, and lavender flowers, with a couple of handfuls of crushed almonds thrown in for flavor. The wine will have the medicinal attributes of the flowers you choose.

CAUTION

Red clover leaf and blossom, along with other herbs that contain coumarin glycosides, including strawberry, blackberry, and raspberry leaves, may form a toxic di-coumarol molecule when improperly dried. Di-coumarol reduces the blood's ability to clot. Pharmaceutical medicine uses it as a powerful anticoagulant. To avoid a potentially serious situation, always be sure to use only fresh or thoroughly dried and properly stored herbs for your wine- or vinegar-making process.

The leaves and seeds of apples, apricots, plums, cherries, and peaches contain a natural form of cyanide, hydrocyanic acid, which is released as that plant part is broken down. Do not add these leaves or seeds to your wine.

MEDICINAL VINEGARS

On the day my daughter was due to be born, I thought I'd get ahead and make a big batch of strawberry wine before things got crazy with a new baby. I gathered strawberries that morning, and by lunchtime I had a 10-gallon crock filled and fermenting. Just when I thought I could sit back and relax, labor started.

Later that day an 8½-pound baby girl was born! She was perfect in every way, and as babies will, she kept us hopping. But the wine turned out to be far from perfect.

In my haste to make the wine, I hadn't sorted out the blemished strawberries, since they had all just been freshly gathered. Then I let the wine sit for several weeks before I finally got around to looking at it. When I took off the cheesecloth, the rapidly fermenting brew had turned to vinegar. My first thought was to throw it all away; it certainly wasn't useful as wine. But curiosity got the best of me and I let the brew finish fermenting. I strained it and decanted off the sediment, and ended up with a five-year supply of the best strawberry vinegar this side of the Mississippi.

It turns out that wine *wants* to sour. This is part of the natural fermentation process. If you add fruit that is not sound, chances are good that bacteria are already present on it. I like making vinegar because I can use up otherwise discarded bruised peaches, apple peelings, and herb stems, thus extending the yield from my harvest.

How to Make Medicinal Vinegars

Since producing my first unplanned batch of vinegar, I've found a few techniques to help ensure a good medicinal vinegar. Following is a recipe to ensure a good batch of vinegar.

Yield: About 2 gallons without sediment

- 2 gallons (8 liters) water
- 1–1½ pounds (400 to 600 g) of herbs
- 2–3 quarts (2–3 liters) fruit
- 1 tablespoon (15 ml) baker's yeast
- ½ cup (125 ml) mother vinegar (see page 20)
- 1 pound (400 g) honey (or other sugar source)

1. Sterilize all the equipment you will use with peroxide (see pages 23–24) or by boiling for ten minutes.

2. Gather your fruits and herbs of choice. Sort and discard any black or obviously molded parts on the fruit. A little bruising or discoloration (brown apple peelings) is okay, however.

3. Since the process of "souring" happens fairly quickly, take one gallon of the water and use it to brew the herbs into a strong tea. Strain and press out excess tea from the plant material. Ultimately this makes a stronger medicinal vinegar than if you first make the vinegar, then add the herbs to vinegar as you would with a tincture. Also, since the herbs are part of the vinegaring process, the resulting acid content is higher, decreasing the chance of spoilage. Add in the other gallon of water, and let cool to room temperature.

4. In a 3-gallon crock or other nonreactive container, combine the 2 gallons of room temperature herb tea, fruit, yeast, mother vinegar, and honey.

5. Cover with three or four thicknesses of clean cheesecloth secured with a rubber band or string. Store in a warm place between 75° and 90°F.

6. A key to vinegar is exposure to air. Remove the cheesecloth and skim off any surface scum that may develop. Then give the brew a good stir (use a nonreactive spoon) once or twice every day for about one week. Skim off any froth that rises from the stirring. Replace the cheesecloth cover when done stirring and skimming.

7. When the fermentation is finished, the bubbling will stop and the brew will no longer be frothy. It will smell and taste sour. This takes about one week. Strain out the fruit. Let settle overnight, covered with the cheesecloth. Remove the cover and slowly pour off the clear liquid from the bottom sediment. Use a turkey baster to carefully get the last bit of clear vinegar out, or set up a simple siphon (see page 70). The bottom sediment may be saved to act as the mother vinegar in your next batch of vinegar.

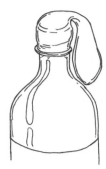

8. Pour the vinegar into the bottles. Slip a small deflated balloon on top to monitor for possible fermentation. When the balloon remains deflated for 24 hours, fermentation has stopped. Now you may safely cork the bottles. Cover the cork with melted beeswax to ensure a proper seal. Label and date your bottles. Store the bottles on their sides.

9. You can use the vinegar right away, but just like wine, the flavors of herb vinegars mellow and blend upon aging. Try to wait at least three months before using, if possible.

Guidelines for Use

Medicinal vinegars can be used in the same ways that the comparable herb wine or tincture would be used. They are excellent for people who are intolerant to alcohol. A tablespoon of honey and a tablespoon of herb vinegar in a cup of water makes a refreshing beverage — hot or cold — to help normalize digestion, restore the acid-alkali balance, and provide energy. They may be freely used internally and externally.

Herbal vinegars are generally not as medicinally potent as their alcohol counterparts, but when made with herbs that nourish the organs such as alfalfa, violet, or red clover, herbal vinegars make a tonic superior to a comparable alcohol tincture. Tonics are a cornerstone to slowly build and maintain a healthy condition. They counteract nutrient deficiency, rebuild vitality, and should be mild and nourishing. Tonics are best taken daily and regularly. Herbal vinegars make a tasty addition to a diet, and their mild nature allows them to be used as a tonic. In fact, I keep taste foremost in mind when putting a vinegar brew together. Lavender, borage, violet, and rose all make sublime vinegars; the more culinary herbs such as ginger and thyme are great, as well.

It is difficult to determine the percentage of acid for homemade vinegars. Commercial vinegar is always 5 to 7 percent, and is strong enough to use as a preservative for pickling. Never use homemade vinegar to pickle vegetables or fresh herbs. The water content of the fresh plants may be just enough to tip the scale too far away from the acid content necessary to preserve the vinegar and prevent botulism from growing. Should you be concerned about a low level of acid, try adding a touch or two of 80-proof alcohol to enhance the preservation.

Although I have often read that medicinal vinegars don't last much longer than six months to a year in storage, I've not found that to be true of well-made homebrewed vinegars. A friend of mine recently used a ten-year-old bottle of homebrewed black-berry vinegar against an intestinal flu that had upset her whole family. She found it very viable indeed.

HIGH-CALCIUM BREW

Vinegar is an excellent medium for carrying calcium into a formula. To make a high-calcium vinegar, incorporate herbs high in this nutrient such as alfalfa, fresh raspberry leaf, and red clover. Another good source is crushed and dried eggshells. Calcium will naturally leach into the vinegar solution until it reaches the saturation point.

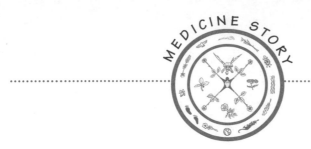

THE RATTLESNAKE MASTER

Once there was a young boy who wanted to learn how to dance with the rattlesnake during ceremony. So he went to the old rattlesnake master and told him of his desire. The old master listened to the boy talk and agreed that the boy could try a test. If he passed, the old man would teach him.

First, the boy had to go to a cave where the rattlesnake lived. He was not to go inside the cave, but instead to draw a circle around himself and sit outside every night from dawn to dusk until a rattlesnake came into his circle. The boy followed his instructions, but sometimes he fell asleep and dreamed about rattlesnakes. Sometimes his legs would cramp and he'd walk around his circle. Sometimes he'd be so bored he wanted to quit. But finally one night a rattlesnake came into his circle.

He went running back to tell the old master. "Good. Now you must learn how to pick up and hold a rattlesnake. After I show you, go back to your circle and try it yourself." And again the boy waited in his circle for many nights until one night he figured out how to call the rattlesnakes to him. The next night he gently touched a rattlesnake. The next night he stroked its back; the night after that, he held its neck; and finally he lifted the rattlesnake up and held it over his head!

He went running back to tell the old master. "Good. Now, go live in the snake's cave for one month." And though the boy was scared, he did as requested. At the end of a month he came back to tell the old man. "Good, but to dance with the rattlesnakes, you must be able to live with them with your eyes closed." So the boy went blindfolded into the rattlesnake's den.

Every day he sat, afraid to move. One night he heard a woman's voice whisper sweetly in his ear. He fell in love with the voice and he asked the woman to marry him. She consented, but said she could only visit her husband at night and he must never take his blindfold off. He agreed. They were married and they had many, many children. The man was happy.

Some days he'd return to his village, but he never told anyone about his wife. Years passed. The villagers wondered where the man went every night. One evening several villagers followed him. That morning when the man came out, the people begged to know what he was doing inside. Finally the man told them about his wife. The people thought it strange that he never saw his wife. They pestered him until he, too, became curious to see his wife.

That night he went to the cave with no blindfold on. When his wife and many children came to play with him, he saw they were all rattlesnakes! He was scared, but then he remembered all the love and joy his rattlesnake family gave him. He decided not to go back to the village, but to stay with his family. He stayed for many years until his wife died and his children were all grown.

He returned to the village an old man. He went to visit his teacher, but the teacher had died many years before. There was no one left who knew how to dance with the rattlesnakes. One villager remembered the old man's strange family. He asked the old man if he could do the dance for the people. And when the time was right, the old man called to one of his children. A rattlesnake came. The snake jumped into his father's arms and they danced together, so happy were they to see each other.

A young boy came out of the crowd when the dance was over. He went up to the old rattlesnake master and said, "Please, can you teach me how to dance with the rattlesnakes?"

As Snake sheds his skin, he throws off the past (death) and continues to live. Thus Snake has been closely associated with healing through all corners of the globe. Hindus, Buddhists, ancient Egyptians, Greeks, and many Native American tribes — the Hopi, Zuni, Cherokee, Seminole, and Sioux — all use snakes in healing ceremonies.

CHAPTER 7

Bittersweets:
Making Syrups and Lozenges

▼▼▼

But they whom truth and wisdom lead
Can gather honey from a weed.

— William Cowper, *Pine-Apple and Bee*, 1779

In my opinion, jams and jellies cry out for a little herbal lift. Plain old strawberry rhubarb jelly is fine, but what if you added a touch of mint? or lavender? Yummm! What if you made a lavender syrup to use as a medicine? Wouldn't that be yummy, too? Perhaps it is simply my sweet tooth speaking, but I get immense satisfaction from sharing my homemade violet syrup on top of a big stack of cattail pollen pancakes with friends. It is the best way I know of to turn another person on to the delights of herbalism. And I can make my family's medicine so tasty that it is easily disguised as food. Thus our food becomes our medicine.

▼▼▼

MAKING MEDICINE PLEASANT TASTING

Syrups disguise the bitter or strong taste of herbs such as dandelion, white pine, raw garlic, and poplar bark. When a syrup is administered straight from the spoon, children don't notice the bitter until after they swallow the medicine. And somehow, the residual sweetness left in the mouth compensates for the bitter taste — enough so that my children, at least, always ask for another spoonful. Try medicinal syrups for anyone who simply cannot or will not tolerate a bitter or strong flavor. Syrups excel at soothing sore throats, coughs, most digestive upsets, and sudden fatigue. However, the high sugar content makes them a poor choice for treating chronic fatigue, nutritive imbalances, or deep-seated chronic disorders such as diabetes.

▲▲▲

HOW TO MAKE A SIMPLE MEDICINAL SYRUP

I'll share with you a process that is by far the easiest way to turn any plain syrup into an epicurean feast. It's good for you, too.

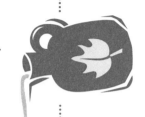

- 1 cup (225 g) water
- ½ ounce (about 2 cups) (250 ml) fresh herb leaf or flower, *or*
- ½ ounce (about ½ cup) (50 ml) herb root or bark (reduce by half if using dried herbs)
- 1 cup (250 ml) honey, maple syrup, rice syrup, or other sweet syrup

1. Bring water to a boil.

2. Remove from heat and add herb leaf or flower. (If you are using root or bark, do not remove from heat, but allow to simmer over low heat until water is reduced by one-half.)

3. Let stand for about half an hour.

4. Strain out herbs, reserving liquid in a saucepan. You now have a very strong cup of tea.

5. Add honey or other syrup to the reserved liquid. Simmer over very low heat on the stove or in an electric warmer that maintains a temperature between 90° and 100°F until most of the liquid is evaporated and the liquid is close in consistency to what the syrup was originally.

6. Bottle, label, and store in a cool dark place or the refrigerator.

FASTER THAN COFFEE

Try starting your day with a cup of instant zing. To make this concoction, add 1 tablespoon of homemade ginger-maple syrup to a cup of hot water. Add a squeeze of lemon. This delicious blend will help kick-start your day without leaving any caffeine jitters to follow.

An Even Simpler Syrup!

Here's a even simpler method for making syrup, using fruit jelly as the sweet base.

1. Make ½ cup (125 ml) of a strong herb tea.

2. Mix tea well with one cup of fruit jelly of your choice. Apple jelly allows the flavor of the herbs to come through the most. Allow it to stand overnight in your refrigerator before using.

This is a good method to use if you're testing a new herb combination and are uncertain about the flavor. I often try out my experiments this way before using them in a more complicated recipe.

You can also make a simple herb jelly by adding ½ cup of fresh, finely chopped herbs and flowers to a fruit jelly. Let stand overnight to give the flavors a chance to blend.

HOW TO MAKE SUGAR-FREE SYRUPS

Low methoxyl-type pectin powders are derived from citrus peels and pulp. They can be used to make jams, jellies, and syrups that rely on calcium to bind and gel rather than sugar (like regular pectin jellies). You can usually find this type of pectin in health food stores: Pomona and Universal are two brand names to look for. When you open the box you'll find two packets, one with pectin, one with calcium. The calcium must be dissolved in water; a small amount of this mix is then added to the recipe.

Selecting Suitable Herbs

To make a syrup using a low methoxyl-type pectin, it's best to use fresh and uncooked herbs. Fresh herbs help give a creamy texture to the recipe, while dried herbs merely seem gritty in comparison. Since the syrup is basically uncooked, delicate flower and herb essences are preserved, plus heat-sensitive vitamins like A and C will not be destroyed. For long-term keeping, however, you will have to store the finished product in the freezer. Try this recipe with all manner of herbs and flowers:

peppermint, rose, red clover blossom, lavender, lemon balm, violet — any pleasant-tasting herb or flower. You can even use hard fruits such as rose hips if you cut the blossom ends off the hips first, then whir the hips in the blender with water until you get a milkshake consistency. Let stand for about 2 hours, then strain out the seeds through a sieve. Use this strained liquid to make your syrup. And of course there are all kinds of delicious fruits you can add to give an extra dimension to the flavor of the herbs Try a lavender and orange juice concentrate blend or apple mint jelly to stimulate digestion. Rose petal, lemon balm, and strawberry is a centering, calming blend. Sweet cherry and lemon thyme syrup is sure to soothe a sore throat and ease coughs. Keep in mind how you will use the syrup as you create your recipes.

> 2 cups (500 ml) of fresh herb or herb-fruit
>   combination
> Lemon juice to taste (add ½ teaspoon [2.5 ml]
>   at a time)
> 1 cup (250 ml) water
> 1 teaspoon (5 ml) methoxyl-type pectin powder

1. Prepare 2 cups of herb or herb-fruit combination. Flower petals like rose or dandelion are bitter at the base. When you gather them, pull the petals up in one hand and clip off the base with a pair of scissors held in the other. This takes about 15 minutes — the same time allotted for the normal coffee break — and is infinitely more relaxing.

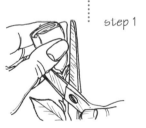

step 1

2. If you wish to add lemon juice, combine it with the fresh herb or petals in a blender. Blend well. It may be necessary to add a little water to get the desired consistency, which should be like a milkshake. Remove from blender and set aside.

3. Bring water to a boil. Put it in the blender and add pectin powder. Blend 1 to 2 minutes, until all powder is dissolved.

4. Add the blended herb mixture to the hot pectin mixture in the blender and process on low for 1 minute.

5. You do not need to add any sugar, but if you want to add sweetener for your own personal taste, add now and blend on low until just mixed.

6. Add ½ teaspoon calcium water (from envelope in pectin mix). Blend again just enough to mix well.

7. Fill three 1-cup freezer-safe containers about two-thirds full and let stand at room temperature for 1 to 2 hours. Store in the refrigerator. This syrup will keep for about three weeks. If, when you go to use it, you discover that it has jelled too much, reheat it and add more water and herb (tea). If it hasn't jelled enough, reheat and add a little more pectin.

To save the syrup longer, so you can open up a jar of this summer sunshine during a January blizzard, store it in the freezer and let it thaw about an hour before serving.

To make jam. By adding a little extra pectin to this recipe, you'll end up with a wonderful no-cook freezer jam.

HOW TO MAKE PASTILLES AND LOZENGES

Pastilles are made with plant powders combined with sugar and a binding agent. Pastilles are dried rather than cooked so the plants retain delicate essential oils. They come in handy for relieving sore throats and mouth sores, or for coating and soothing the stomach for long periods of time. I truly felt that I was free of the tyranny of over-the-counter medicines when I made my first batch of homemade cough drops.

Human names for natural things are superfluous.
Nature herself does not name them. The important thing
is to know this flower, look at its color until the blueness
of it becomes as real as a keynote of music.
— Sally Carrigher, Home to the Wilderness (1973)

Pastilles

This is a great project to do with children. Just put down a protective cloth on and under the table to help with cleanup, then have fun with your herbal play dough.

> ½ cup dried herbs of your choice (try violet or
> rose petal to soothe a sore throat, mint leaf
> or lavender blossom to ease upset stomachs,
> plantain leaf for stubborn mouth sores)
> Maple syrup or honey

1. Pulverize your dried herbs in a mortar, then strain them through a sieve to get a fine powder.

2. Mix the powder with just enough maple syrup or honey to form a ball. It helps to add a mucilaginous plant such as dried marsh mallow root or gum tragacanth (available at many health food stores) to act as a glue. To firm up the consistency, add in more powdered herb ½ teaspoon at a time. Powdered sugar will also absorb excess moisture and sweeten the mixture, and could be added, also ½ teaspoon at a time. Consider adding a pinch of finely chopped balsam poplar buds. The resin helps bind the pastilles, soothe sore throats, and break up congestion, though its flavor is strong.

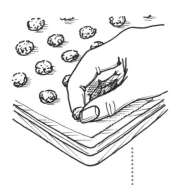

3. When the mixture is firm enough to hold its own shape, mold into small ¼-inch balls. Use right away, or place on a sheet of waxed paper on a cookie sheet and let sit for 12 to 48 hours to harden. Once hard, the pastilles will last longer in the mouth. Wrap each pastille individually to save for future use. Store in a cool dry place.

Lozenges

Making your own cough drops similar to the ones you can buy in the store is easy. It's basically like making an herbal candy.

> 1 ounce (25 g) dried herb, such as thyme, poplar bud, or ginger
> 1½ cups (375 ml) water
> 2 pounds (800 g) refined sugar

1. Combine herbs and water in a saucepan and simmer steadily over low heat for about 10 minutes. Strain liquid into another pan.

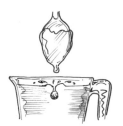

2. Add the sugar to the liquid and bring to a boil. Allow to boil until the mixture reaches 265° to 270°F on a candy thermometer and a few drops form a hard ball when dropped from a spoon into cold water.

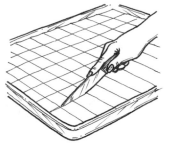

3. Pour mixture into a well-greased 10" x 14" oblong glass or stainless steel cake pan. As soon as it is cool enough to hold its shape, cut it into square lozenges. Wrap each lozenge individually in waxed paper and store in a cool dry place until needed.

Variation. To make a lozenge with a tincture, substitute 1 liquid ounce of the tincture for the dried herb, and reduce the amount of water to ¾ cup. The high temperature will destroy volatile oils such as those found in lemon balm and peppermint. The best way to use a tincture is to simply add it as soon as the sugar mixture is removed from the heat and before it is poured into the pan. When I tried to make a pine sap cough drop, the sap separated out from the sugar, and the method did not work at all. Still, it's worth experimenting with.

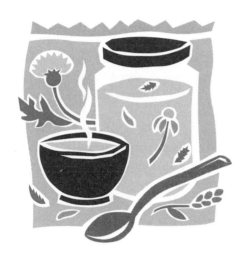

The Mind of Herbalism: Using the Herbs

 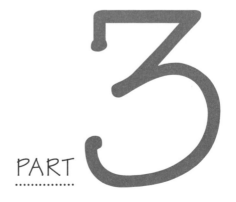

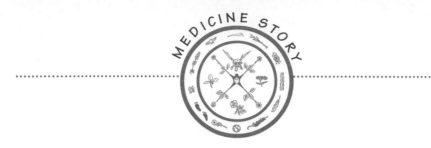

THE NORTH WIND'S GIFT

When the world was still young, the people had only meat and maple sugar to eat. During hard winters, Bukadawin, the Hunger Demon, came close, and the people ate boiled moccasins to keep him away. The men diligently hunted but they returned home with their hands empty and their hearts full of sorrow.

The women could not leave their nursing babies behind to hunt, so they yelled at the men to try again. With each failed hunt, the women grew meaner and the men more sullen. Soon the fighting was heard clear over to the home of the West Wind, and the noise woke Nanaboozhoo.

Curious, he walked to the people's camp. He listened to everyone's complaints and decided to help. But they had to agree that if he tried to help, they would do as he asked, no matter how things might change. The people agreed and Nanaboozhoo went for a walk.

First he walked east until he came to the home of the East Wind. There he found corn. He took some seeds with him, then he walked south. At the home of the South Wind, he found squash. He took some seeds, and then walked west. At the home of the West Wind, he found beans. He took those seeds also, and walked north.

But the home of the North Wind was bitter cold and empty. He walked through the north for six months, finding nothing. Finally, he knew what the north had to offer and he left to return to the people.

The women came running out to meet him. They wept when Nanaboozhoo showed them the seeds because there weren't enough seeds to feed anyone. So Nanaboozhoo threw the seeds on the ground. He told the women to give the seeds water. "These seeds will grow and make more," he told them. "But every six months the North Wind will bring his gift of winter and you will be too busy growing food to argue."

Now both men and women share in the work of providing food. The babies no longer cry, all is peace and quiet, and finally, Nanaboozhoo can get his rest.

Sometimes a trickster, sometimes serious, Nanaboozhoo figures in many of the elder tales of the Anishinaabe. A version of this story is recorded in Althea Helbig's book, Nanaboozhoo, Giver of Life. I first heard it told by Barb Pratt, a Great Lakes storyteller.

CHAPTER 8
Stocking the Home Medicine Chest

▼▼▼▼

Medicine is for the patient . . .
Medicine is for the people . . .
It is not for the profits.

— George Merck

*P*utting together an herbal first-aid medicine chest is a bit like playing the stock market. From a list of companies (the herbs) you choose a few to research and invest in (gathering and preparing), in the hopes that a profit will be made (health). Once one stock (herb) gives you a tidy profit, you are that much more likely to reinvest in it and perhaps expand to try another.

There will be losses, too. Every year I add to my compost pile some of the dried herbs I didn't need because no one broke a bone or had the flu. In fact, many people find that at first they use herbs mostly to treat a cold or earache — acute conditions. But as time goes by, and they start to rely on daily doses of nourishing and gentle herbs, they find that acute conditions happen less frequently, because bones are denser, immunity is stronger, and stress has reduced its hold.

LET NATURE BE YOUR HMO

Just as the stock market changes, so will your family's medicinal needs change. When my children were babies, I relied on big jars of gentle salves and herbs rich in nutrients. When they entered public school, cold prevention became a concern. When sports entered the picture, I stockpiled plants for sprains, cuts, and building stamina.

A good home medicine chest will take into account everyone's needs and have appropriate preparations on hand, ready to use when needed. Since some time and effort goes into this, remember it's also important to store the medicine chest in a cool dark place (and, always, out of the reach of small children) so the medicinals last as long as possible.

BASIC ELEMENTS OF THE
HERBAL HOME MEDICINE CHEST

While there are specialty preparations you'll want to have handy tailored to your family's particular health needs, there are a few standard elements that are useful to have in almost any herbal medicine chest.

ALL-PURPOSE SALVE
This should be a good all-purpose preparation that is antiseptic, speeds healing, and soothes inflamed tissues. Plantain, St.-John's-wort, lavender, thyme, poplar bark, and balsam poplar buds, or combinations thereof, are possible herbs to include in this salve.

ANTIVIRAL TINCTURE
When a virus runs through the house, it can take away everyone's energy — even for those who don't get the bug. I consider a good antiviral tincture or syrup indispensable and essential to have ready to use. St.-John's-wort, raw garlic, honey, red clover, and thyme are all good ingredients for helping the body's immune system ward off invading viruses.

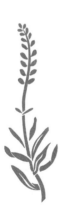

ASTRINGENT WASH
A mild astringent is handy for relieving mild sunburns, stanching bleeding from cuts, soothing insect bites, relieving swollen tissues, and cleansing the face. Dilute rose leaf tincture with 2 parts water and use as a wash; for a stronger action, use walnut leaf tincture.

BALSAM POPLAR BUD TINCTURE
To prevent tape burn, paint the skin with this tincture before applying tape or bandages.

BRUISE AND SPRAIN TREATMENT
Dried plantain leaf, lavender blossom, and poplar bark work well for treating these conditions. Make a tea and lay on the affected area in the form of a poultice to help speed healing and reduce inflammation.

COUGH AND COLD RELIEF

A jar of pine pitch is indispensable for these conditions — use it as a steam pot to break up congestion, or mix it in a salve with peppermint so it can be rubbed on the chest or sore, aching muscles.

A few pieces of dried mallow root are also important to have; chewing on this root helps relieve a sore throat. You could also make peppermint-thyme cough drops, which simultaneously aid the body's immune system and soothe a sore throat. Add mullein, violet, poplar, or garlic to help break up congestion.

DISINFECTANT

Thyme, garlic, lavender, poplar bark, and white pine are all antiseptic by themselves. To disinfect cuts, wash with a tea made from one of these herbs, or make a rubbing alcohol tincture from the herb for a healing disinfectant.

HANGOVER RELIEF

Borage oil is useful for rebuilding the strength after a debilitating illness and as a quick remedy for a hangover taken along with a piece or two of candied ginger. (It also makes an excellent topical oil for dry, itchy skin.)

NAUSEA, INDIGESTION, AND MOTION SICKNESS RELIEF

These conditions can be alleviated by sucking on a few pieces of candied ginger, which is handy to have and stores for a considerable length of time. Also, peppermints or candies made from lavender or catnip may help.

PAIN RELIEF

It can be difficult to be always brewing up teas when in pain. Make a tincture or vinegar to have on hand. Lavender and poplar bark are good for general pain relief. Lemon balm, catnip, and oat straw add a calming dimension as well. Use internally or externally as needed.

FACTORS AFFECTING WHAT'S IN YOUR FAMILY'S MEDICINE CHEST

Ages of members
Personal health needs
Personal goals and temperaments
Lifestyle demands
Access to herbs
Travel requirements and
    interests

SALVE FOR CUTS, SCRAPES, WOUNDS, AND BURNS

When I need more than a simple salve, I turn to white pine pitch — the original liquid Band-Aid. Though it will collect dirt on top, the pitch makes an airtight bandage that is antiseptic underneath. Cover it with a piece of tissue to keep it from sticking to everything. As long as there is no infection, do not remove old

THE MINIMALIST'S MEDICINE CHEST

Herbs can do double and triple duty in your herbal medicine chest. If your resources are limited, choose just one or two multipurpose herbs to begin building your chest: ginger, lavender, peppermint, plantain, poplar, and white pine are all good choices. Each has a wide variety of applications for acute and crisis conditions.

Plantain is my own personal favorite, and it doesn't cost me a cent. When I moved to a place that had no plantain growing nearby, I asked a local market farmer if I could take some plantain from his fields. He was sure I was certifiable, but he even dug and potted the plants for me! But which is crazier: refusing to see the value in what lies under your feet, or purposefully planting weeds in a garden?

I planted the plantain within 10 feet of my door, where it provides a strong contrasting backdrop for my colorful Johnny-jump-ups. Sure, it spreads quickly, but no faster than I use it for medicine and food. So nine months of the year, a valued component of my herbal medicine chest lies right by my doorstep. The other three months, I dig up about a dozen plants and plant them closely in a 2-gallon pot with average soil. Plantain thrives on neglect, but not on poor drainage, so add some sand if your soil has a lot of clay in it. The pot stays by a sunny window through the winter — offering me a year-round supply.

I use plantain much in the way you might an aloe, for poultices for sprains and relief from cuts, mild burns, and swellings. It can be used freely because nature renews the supply, come spring. Plantain happens to be my standard all-purpose remedy. Other people swear by lavender, comfrey, heal-all, nettle, or another plant. Whatever herb you choose is fine; just be sure you have it handy year-round.

pitch; instead, keep applying new fresh pitch until the cut is healed. A salve made from balsam poplar buds will have similar qualities and is good if your skin is sensitive to white pine pitch.

STYPTIC

For bleeding from razor cuts, keep some powdered peppermint leaf on hand — just a sprinkle will stop the bleeding.

Equipment and Supplies

In addition to the herbs and preparations, you'll need the following supplies for applying and administering them and performing other first-aid duties:

- ◆ A glass dropper that can squirt either a few drops of tincture under a tongue or a few drops of healing oil into a sore ear
- ◆ An atomizer for spraying herb teas on the back of sore throats, over large areas of skin, or up stuffy noses
- ◆ An Ace bandage to apply loosely for keeping a poultice in place, or tighter for supporting a sprained limb
- ◆ Fine needle for removing splinters
- ◆ A sharp razor for removing hair around cuts
- ◆ Clean lengths of muslin or gauze in a couple of different sizes for use as handcloths to wash areas with herb teas, or (in larger sizes) to make poultices to lay on the affected area
- ◆ First-aid tape
- ◆ Tissues
- ◆ Pieces of gauze
- ◆ Q-tips
- ◆ Tweezers
- ◆ Small sharp scissors

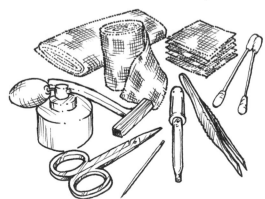

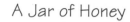

A Jar of Honey

A jar of honey is another valuable first-aid readiness tool to have in the house. A medicine in its own right, honey has powerful antibacterial properties. Pure honey literally sucks the moisture out of bacteria, effectively killing them, while leaving you unharmed. Applied straight it heals external ulcers, wounds, cold sores, genital herpes sores, cysts, and other stubborn-healing sores. Taken internally, it soothes the gastrointestinal tract, calms nerves and spasms, gives energy, and helps the body maintain a stable electrolyte balance (critical when diarrhea, vomiting, or fevers are present). Honey also increases the medicinal effect of natural remedies — especially for the respiratory system. Simply add the indicated medicinal herb dose to a cup of warm water sweetened with honey and sip frequently.

Another technique is to blend equal amounts of honey and herb tincture and use this mixture as needed. Or, mix equal amounts of the freshly chopped herb and honey, let rest for twenty minutes, then apply as needed.

A Beneficial Supply of Yogurt

When illness threatens, stock up on plain yogurt. The beneficial bacteria in yogurt keep the body's digestive system working at peak efficiency. (*Note:* These bacteria are destroyed when sugar or fruit are added, so for medicinal purposes, use only plain yogurt.) Spastic stomachs can usually keep a teaspoon of yogurt down, and that teaspoon will help restore the stomach to a calm condition. A cup of yogurt added to a bath will soothe bladder and vaginal yeast infections, as will a douche made with 2 tablespoons of yogurt in a quart of warm water.

If you must embark on a course of antibiotic treatment, eat a cup of yogurt every day during and for several weeks after treatment. Antibiotics indiscriminately destroy both harmful and necessary bacteria in the body. Eating yogurt reintroduces into the digestive tract beneficial bacteria — the ones without which the digestive process cannot function. Eating plain yogurt will also help prevent renegade yeasts such as candida from multiplying to harmful levels (this is why vaginal yeast infections are so common after a course of antibiotics).

OBSERVE THE FIRST RULE OF FIRST AID

It is a matter of fact that you are assembling your home medicine chest with the hope that you'll never use it — it's your homemade insurance policy. However, the chances are good that you may have to use it, and before you do, be sure to heed the first rule of medicine. Written down by Hippocrates thirty-five hundred years ago, its truth is universally recognized by everyone from ancient ayurvedic Indian practitioners to the modern-day American Medical Association: *First do no harm.*

Assess the Situation Before You Act

Red Cross first-aid training teaches that before you do anything, assess the situation as a whole. Then assess your level of ability to handle it. If it is beyond the scope of your strength, ability, or training, do what you can to stop any imminent dangers that may cause more harm, then go for help. The same holds true at home. Step back and calmly view the situation before embarking on any treatment.

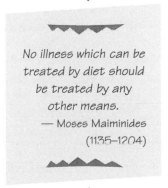

No illness which can be treated by diet should be treated by any other means.
— Moses Maiminides
(1135–1204)

Always aim for the lowest level of intervention whenever possible. The body has a remarkable capacity for self-healing — it wants to get better. Your goal should be to aid the body's desire for health, to encourage its own defense mechanisms to kick into high gear. Strive to be noninvasive. Choose rest, fresh air, and water as the first course of treatment whenever possible. The old doctor's prescription for cold relief, "Take two aspirin and plenty of fluids, go to bed, and call me in the morning," is usually just as effective without the aspirin. The aspirin becomes a psychological crutch, so you feel you are at least doing something to fight the illness, and the doctor doing something to earn his pay. But the water and the rest often do more to stop the cold than the aspirin. Herbs, too, can become a crutch. Use them wisely and sparingly as medicine. Use them freely and liberally as food to build the body's health.

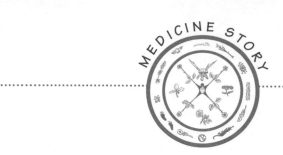

HOW WE GOT STRAWBERRY

There was a time when the People never got sick. But then one day, disease attacked the People. Nanaboozhoo happened to be walking by, and he heard the People crying. He didn't like the noise, so he made "medicine" to help the People get well.

You can imagine how happy the People were. They gave a tremendous honor feast for Nanaboozhoo that lasted for weeks. One evening, a family from a neighboring village asked Nanaboozhoo for help. He was in a pretty good mood, so he made them some medicine. The next day another village came, and then another, and another.

Soon Nanaboozhoo had no time to rest, so he looked about for a helper. His eye fell on Odemin, whose name means "Good Heart." When Odemin could make medicine by himself, Nanaboozhoo left to see what was going on in the rest of the world.

Odemin worked diligently and the People gave him gifts of soft skins and good food. He didn't have to hunt or even clean his own lodge, as long as someone was sick. Soon, Odemin started making the People ill so he could get paid. The People learned to avoid Odemin and his heart grew bitter. No one even looked at him anymore unless they wanted his medicine. So Odemin made a whole family sick, but that wasn't enough. He made whole villages sick, but it still wasn't enough. So he set out to make all the People sick.

Just then, Nanaboozhoo returned. He called up a west whirlwind to snatch up Odemin. The wind spun Odemin until his head came loose, then his arms and his legs. Finally nothing was left but a tiny bitter heart. Just as that, too, was about to disappear, Odemin's heart turned sweet, and he cried out for mercy. He begged Nanaboozhoo for the chance to make amends. Nanaboozhoo took pity on Odemin and had the West Wind release him. Only Odemin's heart remained, and it turned into a strawberry as soon as it touched the ground. Odemin's heart remains small to this day, but it is the sweetest of all the fruits.

I heard this version from Harold and Colleen Katchenago. It's still custom among traditional Anishinaabe mothers to make small heart-shaped strawberry baskets for their babies. First the mother, then the child (as he grows older), places items into the basket to help remember a good deed or brave moment. Ultimately, the basket is buried with the man when he walks west.

CHAPTER 9
Making Herbal Blends

Success is more a function of consistent
common sense than it is of genius.

— An Wang, *Lessons: An Autobiography*

Hopefully, by now you've wondered how some of the herbal recipes were devised. Doesn't it sometimes seem like they must have been just pulled out of thin air? Well, in a way that is true. If you get twenty herbalists in a room and ask them what they most recommend to help ease a cold, I guarantee you will end up with twenty different answers — and all of them will probably be effective. So are there any rules to follow at all? Rules, no; guidelines, yes.

BECOMING A MEDICINE CHEF

Instead of twenty herbalists in a room, imagine there are twenty chefs — and they are making chili. You'd find venison chili, vegetarian chili, chili with white beans, red beans, and no beans, but all of them would be tasty, because they'd be based on the fundamental guidelines of cooking — for instance, for a firm texture and to release flavor into the broth, sauté your vegetables first; but, hey, if you want the vegetables to be soft, put them directly into the pot. A good chef knows what textures and flavors he is aiming for before starting. So does the herbalist.

Types of Illnesses

Illnesses can be put into two categories: chronic and acute. Chronic illnesses involve a weakened or debilitated system. Often many organs or whole body systems are affected. The illness is ongoing and may have been years in development; it is usually serious, and possibly life-threatening. Examples of chronic illnesses are PMS, asthma, arthritis, and diabetes. In contrast, a person with an acute problem is generally healthy, but currently ill or traumatized. Colds, headaches, constipation, and earaches are usually acute. However, if the acute problem becomes frequent or even constant, then it must be treated as a chronic illness, because the system is showing signs of general weakness and debility.

Unfortunately there is no hard and fast rule that defines *chronic* and *acute.* If you have a cold once every three months, most physicians consider the problem acute. If the cold lasts for three months, it would be considered a chronic condition. However, if I get a cold every three months, I consider it a warning that my body is not operating at optimal health, or that my lifestyle and living conditions may need to be reexamined. I ask myself questions such as: Do I simply need to wash my hands more? Slow down? Change my diet?

GUIDELINES FOR DEVELOPING ACUTE-ILLNESS HERBAL FORMULAS

The best way to gain experience and understanding of herbal medicine is to start by treating acute problems. Catnip and peppermint will both calm an upset stomach, but in slightly different ways. The only way to gain a thorough understanding of the difference is to work with each firsthand. In addition, using herbs for acute illnesses builds your confidence in the efficacy of herbal treatment. Once a student of herbalism understands how plantain relieved his bee sting, he becomes more likely to try plantain for poison ivy, or constipation. Eventually the student will understand how plantain might be used to treat a chronic condition such as recurring PMS or an ulcer. Then the student is on the road to mastering plantain.

Beginning Blending

Once you understand the action of two or more herbs, you are ready to start to make your own herbal blends. We blend herbs when we want an action that is generally not found within a single plant. For instance, strawberry leaves gathered before the plant blossoms help promote circulation, while peppermint brings warmth to an area. Put them together and you have a blend that warms cold fingers and toes from the inside. You can actually feel the blood rush to your hands and feet after drinking a cup of this tea. It is, then, excellent for frostbite and cold sensitivity.

Using herbal blends gives you greater flexibility in developing a treatment targeted to the exact condition being experienced, and exponentially increases the range of possible remedies you can address with the plants available to you. Even if you have only four plants available — say, ginger, mallow, poplar, and borage — you still have eleven possible herbal combinations. Using different combinations of these four plants will allow you to tailor the formula to specific needs. If you have a fever, you may wish to combine ginger's warmth with poplar's ability to reduce aches and inflammations. If you have an upset stomach, the action of ginger and mallow will be more soothing to the digestive system, but if your energy is low, the energizing combination of ginger and borage would be a better choice.

The Fewer Herbs Used, the Better the Combination

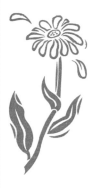

The tendency is to think that if a two-herb combination gives me all this flexibility in tailoring a formula to address a specific condition, how about three-, four-, and five-herb formulas? What if I combined all twenty-five of the herbs listed in this book, then what? Wouldn't that be a formula that would help any acute condition, no matter what? Unfortunately, no. The more herbs used in a formula, the more difficult it becomes to balance their different properties. Each herb acts on its own as well as in relation to the other herbs. So it is actually preferable to use the smallest number of herbs possible in any medicinal formula.

More Difficult Blending

Once you start putting together more than two herbs, there are some guidelines on proportions of various herbs to help you build your formula.

Address the problem. More than half of the blend should address the specific problem. Often in acute ailments, you are looking for an eliminative action (to increase the output of phlegm, urine, stool, sweat, or pus). This may come from one herb or a combination of several herbs with a similar action. For example, for a spring tonic, dandelion or burdock could be used separately or in combination. Either way, the final amount should be anywhere from 50 to 75 percent of the formula.

Soothing qualities. About 10 percent of the blend should be a soothing herb. The herb could be mucilaginous (such as plantain or marsh mallow); soothing to the digestive tract (such as lavender, oats, or catnip); or calming (such as lemon balm, oats, catnip, or rose petal). I always include more of the mucilaginous herbs when I'm using internal eliminative herbs (diuretics, expectorants, or laxatives).

Nurturing qualities. About 10 percent of the blend should be a nurturing, or building, herb. The body needs extra reserves of minerals and vitamins when fighting an ailment. Help by adding a nourishing herb such as violet or dandelion greens, alfalfa or plantain seeds, rose hips or oat straw.

Stimulating qualities. About 5 percent should be a warming, or stimulating, herb, such as ginger, garlic, lavender, peppermint, or thyme. These help kick the body's innate healing process into high gear and enhance the action of the primary medicine. I find that the strongly nutritive herbs, such as alfalfa and borage, may initiate this response also, and are safer to use for borderline chronic-acute conditions.

KEEPING BLENDED FORMULAS SIMPLE

At first glance, it may seem that every formula you devise will have to have at least four different herbs. But this is not so. Every individual herb has several different properties. Ginger and peppermint are both stimulants that also aid digestion. Oats and green oat straw not only calm nerves, but also soothe and nourish the entire digestive system. Lavender is a warming herb that calms nervous tension as well. Keep your formulas as simple as possible and they will have more flexibility in their applications; therefore, they are more likely to be used.

GUIDELINES FOR DEVELOPING CHRONIC-ILLNESS HERBAL FORMULAS

A person with a chronic disorder is in a generally weakened condition. Herbs with strong actions should be avoided, as they may place too much stress on the system. Each formula should be tailor-made for the individual, reevaluated regularly, and changed during the course of the treatment as the person shows improvement or other symptoms begin to manifest themselves. Because of this, all people using herbal therapy for chronic ailments must take an active role in their personal healing. Since mild herbs are used, the course of the treatment is usually for an extended period of time, and a strong level of commitment is necessary.

May the Force Be with You: Begin with What You Eat

Diet plays an important role in chronic disorders. It is a fact that as people use more prepackaged and highly processed foods, their overall health declines. A degenerative diet produces degenerative health. The typical Western diet produces high numbers of degenerative diseases such as arthritis, diabetes, osteoporosis, allergies, heart disease, and cancer. Even the "fresh" produce bought in the supermarket is anything but. It has been picked green, stored, shipped, stored again, displayed, bought, and then stored again — often as long as a month before you eat it. It is not easy to find access to vital food.

Perhaps this is why we have wheat grass devotees and *kombu-cha* drinkers. These are living foods. So is plain yogurt, whole grains (until they are ground), and beans (sprout them yourself for greater vitality). We can seek out the organic sellers of unfiltered honey, raw milk, and fertile eggs. It is work; it does take effort. But being ill steals your efforts faster.

VITAL FOOD

Vital food has the capacity to sustain and nurture life. It is still alive (or very recently alive) as we eat it. When considering whether the food you're eating is vital, ask yourself: If I put this bean into the ground, would it sprout? Could this carrot grow? Does it contain living beneficial bacteria like in yogurt or miso or fresh natural enzymes like in raw honey and milk? Just when was this grain ground?

The self-perpetuating cycle of life: Life casts off death
and remains vital by devouring life.

An ancient Hindu symbol shows a serpent devouring its own tail. It represents life eating life — life must eat itself in order to stay alive. For this, we can look to the vitality in our food, and let its life-force become the life in our bodies that creates balance and health, thereby completing the circle of life. Using fresh-gathered plants as food plays a dramatic role in rebuilding health.

Trust in the Force

Since only mild herbs are used to treat chronic conditions, the results will be mild as well. Indeed, changes *should* be gradual, and result in more energy and lighter spirits at first. Since there may be no noticeable relief of the symptoms, many people are inclined to believe a treatment is not helping and give up after a week or so. But remember, you are not treating the symptoms; you are trying to improve the health of the system as a whole. Only when the person's constitution becomes stronger may stronger herbs be employed. This is usually a gradual process; the ideal course is to gradually add small doses of these stronger herbs during treatment. If at any time stronger symptoms of the disease manifest themselves, the herbal treatment should be changed.

Seek Balance

Chronic diseases often result from long-term imbalance in the body. So when you are developing an herbal formula, it is especially important not to bring in more imbalance. The herbs chosen should balance or cancel each other out. If, for example, a mild laxative such as walnut leaf is used, it could be balanced with a mild astringent such as rose petal. If garlic is used to help lower blood pressure, its heat could be counterbalanced with cooling dandelion leaf. In fact, steamed dandelion leaves in a little garlic and vegetable broth is one tasty way to have your medicine and eat it, too.

CREATING YOUR PERSONAL HERBAL FORMULAS

Remember that simply by combining two herbs, you have created a formula. And the fewer herbs you use, the closer to ideal the formula is. You can now see, given the blending guidelines on pages 100–102, why it can be difficult to pare your choice of herbs for a particular formula down to only two or three. I find, however, that if I keep the purpose of the formula foremost in my mind, the task is easier. It is also easier to blend herbs for an individual rather than an ailment. It is easier yet to blend herbs for yourself.

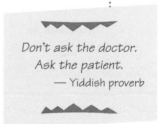

Don't ask the doctor.
Ask the patient.
— Yiddish proverb

Begin with Your Own Habits and Lifestyle

You know yourself best of all. No matter how many charts, forms, or interviews any medical healer may conduct with you, there will be much undiscovered territory. For example, before deciding whether to take a cup of tea, a tincture, an herbal bath, or a pill, each of us must consider how busy our day is, where we are, our personal preferences, and the availability of the herbs — each and every time.

What if you live in the city, or a rural area? Doesn't that affect your choices? What if you hate the taste of garlic, or don't have the patience to crack walnuts? How much effort do you really want to put into gathering, preparing, storing, and using herbs? Only you can answer these questions. Take the time to ask them, and be honest in your answers. And remember, you are already an expert about yourself.

Start Small and Experiment

Keep your batches small at first. In fact, it is a good idea to store your herbs singly. Then blend them as you use them. This gives you greater opportunity to explore the individual nuances of each blend. If I am putting together a blend for the first time, I open each jar of herb and set it on the table. I take a moment to take stock of where my energy level is at: Am I tired or wide-awake? Calm or anxious? Then I breathe deeply of the combination of the herbs (still in their jars) for a minute or so, and take stock of any changes in my body, mind, and spirit.

When you inhale an herb you take into your body its aroma-therapeutic essences. You gather and note your impressions of scent, flavor, action, balance, and use. And though this process may not tell you all the medicinal attributes of a formula, it certainly helps predict your personal affinity for the blend. Because if you don't like a blend — if it doesn't set right with you (and I'm not talking just flavor here) — you won't use it.

Then, if you decide to use the blend, make a small batch first. First try it in a simple way: as a cup of tea, a foot soak, or a bath. These methods will allow you to determine the action of the herb more directly. If possible, try your formulas during different times to see how they affect you — for example, try them during times of high physical activity as well as times of high mental activity.

EXPERIENCE IS THE BEST TEACHER

To gain innate understanding of how a simple herb or formula made from simples affects you individually, you may want to take the herb during a brown rice day or half-day fast (unless an existing medical condition precludes this). Since the effect of brown rice on the body is neutral, the medicinal actions of the formula can be readily discerned. Brown rice contains the nourishment necessary to help keep your energy level stable.

CHAPTER 10

Symptoms and Remedies:
An A–Z Guide to Treating What Ails You

Ad sanitatem gradus est novisse morbum.
(When the illness is known, it is half cured.)

— Latin proverb

Now that you know the healing capacity of the herb and how to prepare it for use, you are halfway to being ready to use that herb for a home remedy. Before you begin, however, take the time to understand the characteristics of the illness or condition. The best herbal remedy in the world is no help when used inappropriately. The following general guidelines will help you learn how to use your herbal remedies safely and effectively. Neither the list of ailments nor the guidelines are fully comprehensive. There are many other complaints herbs can be used for; these only represent some of those easiest treated at home. You'll notice that I include several different choices of remedies using the twenty-five herbs discussed in this book. When possible, try the gentler course of treatment first; fresh air, water, good food, and rest. Select the remedy that has the most relevant action, and that you have available.

Remember that herbal remedies should not be used as a substitute for consultation or treatment by a duly licensed health care professional. When in doubt, seek advice, especially if you are currently taking a pharmaceutical prescription. Many physicians realize that an increasing number of patients are using herbs, and they will at the very least appreciate your being up front about what you are taking. Many can advise about possible herb-drug interactions, and some may even support your efforts to take an active role in your health.

ALLERGIES (HAY FEVER)

Over-the-counter allergy medicine is one of the pharmaceutical industry's best moneymakers. These medications excel at suppressing symptoms, but do little to help the body build a balanced defense system. In fact, they can start a vicious cycle of dependency, ultimately pushing you into seeking even more expensive prescription treatment.

Herbal treatment of allergies involves a three-step process:

1. Avoid exposure. Try to avoid exposure to the allergen whenever possible.

2. Build your natural defenses. Work to build a balanced defense system by using daily doses of fresh, mineral-rich herbs before the allergies manifest themselves. People have found relief from an entire hay fever season by eating abundant amounts of violet greens, dandelion greens and root, along with burdock root in the early spring. These herbs also help the liver break the allergens down into harmless compounds. Keep the regimen up as the season progresses with fresh alfalfa, plantain greens, red clover, and rose hips.

Another old-time remedy is to eat comb honey in four-day cycles several weeks before the hay fever season begins. Local comb honey is considered best. This has varying results, but is so pleasant that it is certainly worth a try.

3. Ease the symptoms. Use steam pots for inflamed stuffy sinuses. Put a handful of decongestant herbs such as mullein, peppermint, and white pine needles into a pot of boiling water. Remove from the heat, drape a towel over your head and the pot, then breathe deeply for several minutes. Take

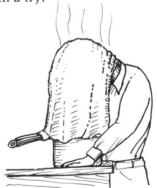

HERBAL ANTIBIOTIC PREPARATIONS

◆ **Garlic-infused wine.** Chop garlic, cover with wine, and let rest for several hours.

◆ **Garlic honey.** Prepare as above, substituting honey for wine. Excellent for cold sores.

◆ **Garlic lemonade.** Prepare as above, substituting honey lemonade for wine, to make a refreshing beverage.

◆ **Garlic water.** Crush 2 large cloves in a quart of water. Let sit for about 6 hours. This may be used on sensitive areas, and internally as a douche.

the herb water from the steam pot and use it as a nasal spray if you are working or traveling.

Bathe sore, irritated eyes with an infusion of plantain leaf, or bruise the fresh leaves and place them directly on the eyelids for several minutes.

ANTIBIOTICS (Herbs to use during and after a course of treatment)

Antibiotics are overprescribed in this country. This is partly the fault of the patient who demands them, and partly the fault of the current medical system that allots only fifteen minutes for a doctor's visit, which leaves little time for patient education. Though the decision to prescribe antibiotics rests with the physician, the responsibility to take them rests with the patient. There are few practices as harmful to your health as taking an antibiotic treatment only until the symptoms disappear — always finish the course of treatment once started.

I heartily recommend you question your doctor if he prescribes antibiotics. Remember the doctor is giving advice, not a law set in stone, and assumes you know nothing. I ask the physician to rate the seriousness of the problem on a scale of one to ten. That helps me understand the situation. I also make it clear that I would prefer to use rest and simple therapies first. Once doctors understand that I am willing to take an active role in healing, I find most will go so far as to offer advice on how to work with alternative treatments — as long as they feel the ailment is not life-threatening.

When a physician gave my three-month-old son's earache a five on the scale, he helped me decide to treat the earache with home remedies first, and to use antibiotics only if the condition worsened. However, when I developed an abscess while nursing and in just a few hours found the whole breast red and inflamed, while my temperature spiked quickly up to 103°F, I was relieved to have the option of antibiotics available.

Replenish healthy bacteria. Antibiotics act indiscriminately in the body, killing off both harmful and beneficial bacteria. Our body relies on certain helpful bacteria to aid digestion and keep other harmful bacteria at bay. To keep a constant replenishment of healthy bacteria in your body, eat at least one 8-ounce serving of plain yogurt every day during and

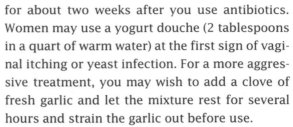

A normal healthy person has so many bacteria in his body that were he to suddenly become invisible, every detail down to the eyelashes could be distinguished by the bacteria present just on the surface of the skin.

for about two weeks after you use antibiotics. Women may use a yogurt douche (2 tablespoons in a quart of warm water) at the first sign of vaginal itching or yeast infection. For a more aggressive treatment, you may wish to add a clove of fresh garlic and let the mixture rest for several hours and strain the garlic out before use.

Herbs to aid digestion. Antibiotics disturb digestion. Drink teas that soothe and aid the process such as mallows, plantain, and catnip; or combine ginger, peppermint, thyme, or lavender with mallow root. Sweeten freely with honey.

Herbs for rebuilding strength and immunity. After a course of antibiotics is finished, help rebuild your body's immune system with herbs that enhance its functioning. Especially beneficial are raw garlic and thyme, taken in six-day cycles (allow one day of rest from treatment).

The combination of illness and antibiotic leaves your body depleted of nutrients and vitality. Rebuild your strength quickly with dandelion and violet salads or soups, morning oatmeal, alfalfa or plantain seeds or sprouts sprinkled on your food, young plantain leaves lightly sautéed in walnut oil, or cups of nourishing herb teas such as oat straw, borage, red clover, strawberry leaf, and alfalfa.

ANTISEPTICS

Nature generously provided us with thousands of plants with antiseptic value. Antiseptic action from a whole plant is generally milder than that from the plant's essential oil, and so is better to use for minor conditions or as a preventative. For quicker, more immediate action, the essential oil may be used (usually in a diluted form). I strongly suggest you reference a book on essential oils (see page 157) before use, as they are extremely potent substances.

Burdock. Decoct the roots and/or seeds for a skin wash that is unparalleled in its ability to heal chronic skin disorders such as boils, cysts, open ulcers, and scaling eczema. Lay the herb on as a poultice and wrap with a warm towel for such stubborn-healing sores.

Garlic. Nature's broad-spectrum antibiotic, antifungal, antiparasitic, antiprotozoan, and antiviral agent. Research shows that raw garlic extracts act more effectively in rats than the common antibiotic tetracycline! Garlic owes its incredible powers to a compound called *allicin,* which is tricky stuff. You have to chop into it to release its action. Also, the allicin is highly unstable; left alone, half of it will degrade within three hours at room temperature, and it will all nearly vanish within twenty-four hours. Heat completely breaks down allicin within twenty minutes. Forget about using garlic capsules — their allicin component is negligible (although they do contain compounds effective in lowering cholesterol).

Honey. For a quick dressing, smear the affected area with pure honey. Honey is a powerful antibiotic in its own right. Avoid applying straight honey on dry, chapped, or flaky skin, as it may worsen the condition.

Lavender. A useful wound herb, lavender's name comes from the Latin *lavare,* "to wash." Lavender tea is excellent for all manner of external skin ailments, as a mouthwash, and in an ointment for mild burns, cuts, and scrapes.

Poplar bark. Though its antiseptic action is comparatively mild, poplar combines anti-inflammatory action and pain relief for a triple-power-packed punch. Poplar works best in herbal combinations such as poplar-plantain to heal bruises quickly, poplar-marsh mallow for gastric inflammations, and poplar-garlic for inflamed bug bites and scrapes.

Thyme. Thyme is a favorite internal remedy for infections and inflammations. Its active compound, thymol, is exceptionally antiseptic. Add fresh thyme to soups and stews during illness, as well as drinking the medicinal tea. Thyme tea makes an excellent gargle for strep throats, and can also be added to the bath and used in compresses and footbaths.

White pine sap. Apply the sticky sap right onto cuts, scrapes, burns, and wounds for instant pain relief, antiseptic action, and a bandage. Excellent to use in the field, especially over large scrapes. No white pine tree handy? I have found that the extruded resins from white and black spruce; red, jack, pitch, and yellow pines; tamarack; and the north woods favorite, balsam fir, to be just as effective.

Other herbs. Those that demonstrate antiseptic activity include gingerroot, lemon balm leaf, mullein leaf and flower, peppermint leaf, rose petal, St.-John's-wort leaf and flower, violet leaf, and walnut leaf.

APHRODISIACS

Thyme. European tradition called for young men to drink thyme tea before they were wed to increase their sexual interest — which was, perhaps, more important in the days of arranged marriages. I know several men who wholeheartedly believe that this formula works and imbibe thyme tea (or thyme honey) freely and regularly, to their satisfaction.

Lavender. Massage your partner with a lavender massage oil. Lavender has traditionally been considered a sensual herb; simply inhaling its essential oil has been shown to excite penile erection and maintain it for longer periods of time.

Rose. This flower has always been associated with love. Its subtle action lies in the essential oil of the flowers; a simple bouquet of rose and lemon balm leaves placed in a room will help dispel nervous anxiety and gladden the heart. Sipping rose petal wine also stirs the heart, but be careful, for — as they say — alcohol increases the desire while stealing the ability.

Other herbs. In traditional Chinese medicine, burdock root has a reputation for increasing sexual desire; in the Middle East, alfalfa was said to make both man and horse virile.

ASTRINGENTS

Use an astringent wash to tighten the skin and mucous membranes, and to check excessive body secretions. They are useful for checking bleeding, tightening and relieving hemorrhoids, and treating swollen tonsils, varicose veins, and diarrhea.

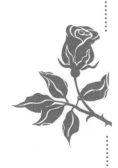

Many astringents are high in tannin, the substance that makes your cup of black tea leave a dry aftertaste in the mouth. Rose leaf, poplar bark, raspberry leaf, and blackberry leaf are strong astringents. Use them as gargles, washes, lotions, teas, tinctures (generally stronger than teas and usually diluted with water), ointments, douches, and mouthwashes.

BACK PAIN

Much lower back pain is temporary and nothing seems to cure it better than rest. If there's any inflammation of the area, apply cold packs. Then, after the swelling subsides, heat may be used to keep the muscles relaxed. Most doctors recommend that you not stay down constantly with minor back pain, as the muscles can weaken and further complicate the problem.

St.-John's-wort. This herb has a direct healing action on nerve tissue and is sometimes nicknamed *chiropractor in a bottle.* Gently rub it onto the affected area of the back or neck for extra healing relief. Drink doses of St.-John's-wort to help heal the nerves from within.

Tea. Invariably, when my back hurts, I have been doing too much running around for everyone but myself. It is my body's way of making me take the time to slow down, calm, and relax (whether I think I can or not). Drinking lemon balm or rose petal tea helps add the dimension of taking care of myself back into my routine.

Poplar bark. Drink infusions of poplar bark to ease pain and inflammation. But be careful — pain is nature's way of telling you to rest. Pain-diminishing herbs are best used when you know you will be taking it easy, not to allow you to keep on going until real damage is done.

BLEEDING, CUTS, AND SCRAPES

To control bleeding from a wound, elevate the injured part and, with a clean cloth, press directly on the wound. Keep pressing until the bleeding stops. If the bleeding is serious, do not take the pressure away to brew a cup of tea or powder an herb. Instead maintain pressure and seek medical attention.

White or black walnut bark tea. This will act as a styptic to stanch the flow of blood from a cut. Compresses of the strong tea are most effective.

Peppermint leaf. Finely powdered, this will immediately help clot blood; it's especially helpful to control nosebleeds and razor cuts. For nosebleeds, tilt head back and pinch the nose firmly until the bleeding stops. Use only small amounts of the powdered leaf. I remember being hesitant to try this, worried that it would sting or, by adding "'debris" to the cut, make it worse. It does neither, as long as the peppermint is finely powdered. Try it on a small paper cut first if you are unsure.

Red raspberry leaf. This can be drunk during pregnancy and delivery to help prevent uterine hemorrhaging.

Astringent herbs. Herbs such as lavender, rose, and inner poplar bark made into an infusion are excellent for washing the debris from scrapes.

Garlic wine. See instructions for making this on page 108; it will simultaneously cleanse and prevent infection in wounds and cuts. To protect area after cleansing, apply a paste of garlic honey over areas larger than a quarter, or white pine sap over areas smaller than a quarter as a protective bandage.

St.-John's-wort oil. This will help stimulate the nerve endings for rapid healing. Be sure the cut is clean, as the new skin may grow over dirt and infection.

BOILS AND ABSCESSES

Applications of warm washcloths may be all that is needed to bring a boil or abscess to a head. If it occurs in the breast of a nursing woman, have her continue nursing or expressing milk during treatment, and monitor for signs of mastitis. (These include fever, the area becoming hot to the touch, and nauseous flulike symptoms. Medical treatment may be necessary.)

Honey. This is one of the oldest and simplest remedies for stubborn boils. It can be applied directly to raise the boil; for best results, leave on overnight.

Plantain. Help bring a boil to a head by applying freshly bruised (or chewed) plantain leaf or root to the area. Bind with a cloth and repeat several times a day. Mullein root, mallow root, and violet leaf may be used in a similar manner.

Thyme. Dip a cloth in a cup of strong, warm thyme tea. Apply this compress for ten to fifteen minutes at a time, remoistening the cloth in the warm tea as it cools. Do this several times a day as necessary.

BRUISES

Soothing herbs. Compresses, poultices, or fresh herbs can be simply applied directly to the skin. Use soothing herbs such as lemon balm, mallow root, plantain, violet, walnut leaf, and borage leaf. Add the strong tea to a bath for larger areas. Ointments made from any of these soothing herbs can be spread on afterward to speed healing and relieve discomfort.

Burdock. Drink burdock root tea to help the lymph system heal the bruise from within. You can also wrap the area with large fresh burdock leaves to cool and reduce swelling. Replace with fresh leaves as they become warm and dry.

Mullein. Applications of mullein flower oil are traditionally used in many European households to speed healing and ease painful bruising. The oil is safe enough to use around sensitive areas such as eyelids, mouth, nose, and genitals.

Vinegar. Apply hot or cold compresses of vinegar. Especially helpful are vinegars made with astringent fruits such as blackberry, raspberry, and rose, as they will also help reduce swelling and inflammation.

BUG BITES AND STINGS

For a natural bug repellent, make a smudge by tying together dried lavender, peppermint, mullein, or catnip into a tight cylindrical bundle with thin wire. Light the bundle and keep it nearby. The smoke from the smudge masks your scent and the CO_2 being released with your breath, making it difficult for insects to find you.

If you're out in the field, treat any bites or stings immediately. Honeybees and some wasps leave their stingers behind. Gently scrape them off. Do not pull, as you'll actually release more poison into the sting. Plants such as plantain, mullein, violet, and red clover blossom soothe quickly. Actually, the chlorophyll found in any nonpoisonous green plant will provide relief. Simply rub the juice from the freshly crushed (or chewed) plant on the area. Keep it dirt-free to prevent infection.

Once at home, clean the site well with an antiseptic herb wash such as lavender or thyme, and apply an ice pack to reduce swelling.

For anyone with a large number of insect bites and stings, help the body break down the toxins with herb teas such as oat straw, dandelion root, red clover, and burdock root.

A smudge bundle is a natural bug repellent.

BEWARE BUG BITE ALLERGIES

Always watch for signs of an allergic reaction. About one person in two hundred has a latent severe allergic response because their immune system has been sensitized by a previous bite. A subsequent bite — even years later — may trigger a response that leads to shock and possibly death. Emergency medical intervention is required when:

◆ There is swift localized swelling
◆ The person was stung in the throat or the mouth
◆ Swallowing or breathing becomes difficult
◆ The face, lips, eyes, or tongue swells
◆ Nausea, vomiting, stomach cramps, or diarrhea occurs
◆ The person is dizzy or collapses

BURNS AND BLISTERS

Do not try to treat third-degree burns, burns over a large area of the body, or chemical or electrical burns at home. Instead, stabilize the person, monitor for shock, and arrange transport or emergency medical treatment immediately. I have, however, treated severe second-degree burns when necessity demanded it.

First, assess the situation and remove the person from any further danger. If it is a chemical burn, keep flushing the skin with cold running water until well after the pain has stopped. Keep foremost in mind the importance of not damaging the skin any further, and keep the burn as clean as possible. Clean the area of any debris or dirt very gently — do not break any skin or blistered areas. For first- and mild second-degree burns, immediately place the area in cold water to ease the pain, as long as the skin is not broken.

Vitamin E. There has been much research done showing the efficacy of vitamin E oil to heal burns. The oil works in three ways: It rapidly heals damaged nerve endings; it attracts dead skin cells that are being sloughed off naturally, acting as a natural skin graft; and it acts as an antioxidant to prevent infection.

Salve. A combination of St.-John's-wort and poplar made into a salve with vitamin E (rose hip seeds are a good source) will add the dimension of pain and inflammation relief and nerve fiber rejuvenation to a remedy. Smear the area liberally with the salve. Bandage, changing the dressing two or three times a day until signs of healing are obvious. New skin may grow back fused together, so wrap digits individually. Monitor for any signs of infection, and seek treatment if the area shows any signs of worsening.

White pine sap. If you're in the field, you can re-create the effects of the salve with white pine sap. The Ojibway always made sure there was a white pine tree (or balsam fir, tamarack, or spruce) right next to the fires in their maple sugar camps to heal the inevitable burns and blisters. Reserve straight white pine sap for field use or smaller burns, as it will attract a lot of dirt to its surface. This is fine for small areas, as the dirt can be contained; as the old sap falls off of larger areas, though, the possibility of contaminating the burn increases. Do not remove the old sap; instead, simply cover the area with new sap until healing is complete. When we were camping, my two-year-old son placed his palm on a hot woodstove. His moderate to severe second-degree burns healed without complications or scars, using only constant applications of white pine sap. I've had similar results using balsam fir or balsam poplar bud resins.

DO HERBAL SALVES HEAL?

Once, out of curiosity as to whether it was the salve itself that heals or the herbs in the salve, I experimented on a case of diaper rash. On one area, I applied a plain jojoba and beeswax salve; on the other I used the same plain salve as a base, but augmented it with infused plantain and lemon balm. Would I surprise you if I said that the herbal salve healed overnight, while the plain salve took a week to heal? I hope not, because that's what happened.

Tea. Give the burned person plenty of fluids. A tea made from poplar and lemon balm will help calm the patient and provide a further measure of pain relief.

Salves for sunburn. For sunburn and mild burns, cool the area with cold water or a vinegar splash, then apply a soothing and healing salve. Salves from violet, poplar, rose, lavender, red clover, or plantain will prove helpful.

Mallow root. Cook mallow root until the liquid resembles a gooey egg white, allow to cool, and apply to large areas of minor sunburn. Once the sunburn starts to heal, mix this with an equal amount of thick oat water for relief from itching.

Make oat water as you would any other simple tea, using 1 ounce of rolled oat as the herb to 1 quart of water. Strain and cool before using.

CHAPPED SKIN

Oats. Fill a muslin bag with oats, tie it, and add it to your bathwater; or rub it over the chapped area several times daily.

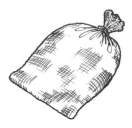

Healing salve. Spread a soothing, healing salve over the affected area. Add extra beeswax, lanolin, coconut oil, or cocoa butter, for a thicker, longer-lasting salve. Infused plaintain and lemon balm are healing additions (see box on page 117). Other helpful herbs to use are violet leaf, mullein leaf or root, mallow leaf or root, red clover blossom, and St.-John's-wort leaf. Avoid applying honey or white pine pitch to chapped skin — it will dry the skin further.

COLDS AND COUGHS

Mild herbal tea. One of the nice things about herbal teas is the amount of water they encourage you to drink. I have quite literally drunk colds away. I'll brew up a pot of whatever mild and nourishing herb I have and drink, drink,

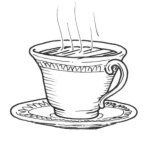

drink . . . as much as a quart an hour if I feel really foul. Make the tea pleasant to taste, rather than medicinal, so you can drink large amounts. Try teas made from rose hips or petal, alfalfa, borage leaf, catnip, dandelion, fresh lemon balm, peppermint, red clover, strawberry leaf or flower or fruit, violet leaf or flower . . . you get the idea.

Baths. Combine the previous tea therapy with hot foot- or full baths of ginger or peppermint to induce perspiration and eliminate body toxins. This can also reduce head congestion by drawing blood away from the head and into the feet.

Mullein leaf. An infusion of fresh or dried mullein leaf is the prime remedy for easing bronchial complaints, hacking or spastic coughs, and lung complaints. To offset its tannin content, boil the leaves in milk for 10 minutes, then strain through a cloth to remove the tiny leaf hairs.

Some people prefer to smoke mullein and substitute mullein leaf for tobacco in hand-rolled cigarettes or light the leaves in a stone dish and inhale the smoke. Smoking mullein has the same effect as drinking a mullein infusion, only the action is faster. And as with any remedy, the faster the action, the greater chance for harm: in this case, though the medicine is healing, the method used (smoking) may be irritating. However, I have successfully used mullein smoke to instantly stop dangerous whooping cough spasms and mild asthma attacks, and I certainly prefer it to the side effects that come from using the medication in over-the-counter and prescription inhalers.

Honey. Take a teaspoon of fresh honey for immediate relief from irritating tickle coughs. Make a honey syrup from violet blossom, borage leaf, crushed garlic clove, mallow root, plantain leaf, red clover blossom, thyme, or white pine needle. All have expectorant or emollient properties.

Garlic. Garlic's reputation for healing bronchial and lung complaints is well deserved. I have seen it cure chronic bronchitis that antibiotics could not touch. Adding a fresh clove of garlic a day to the diet can prevent asthma attacks and reverse that disease's deadly downward spiral. Eat a sprig of parsley or dandelion leaf afterward to help control garlic's odor.

Pine. Pour a quart of boiling water over a good handful of fresh pine needles, place a towel over your head and the pine tea, and breathe deeply of its vapors to break up congestion quickly. When finished, strain and drink the beverage to get high doses of vitamins C and A to further speed your recovery. Adding a little lemon and honey will make the beverage more enjoyable.

For herbal therapies that help the body's immune system combat cold viruses, see the section on flu prevention.

CONSTIPATION

Constipation is usually caused by not eating enough fruits, vegetables, or foods with natural fiber, or by lack of exercise. The safest remedy may be as simple as drinking several glasses of water and enjoying a walk.

Strawberry. This fruit has a mild laxative effect, and is especially useful when the constipation is due to excessive meats or fats in the diet.

Mullein. Mullein tea made with milk will help a person pass hard stools easier because of its demulcent and emollient properties.

Greens. Intensely green leaves are slightly laxative to many people. Add servings of fresh or steamed violet leaf, dandelion greens, or plantain leaf to the diet. This has the added benefit of replacing possible lost nutrients.

Honey. This also has a slight laxative effect.

Plaintain. Pour a cup of boiling water over 1 tablespoon of coarsely ground plantain seeds. Let sit for 20 minutes and drink, without straining, just before bedtime. This is an excellent laxative for more persistent constipation, or constipation from pregnancy, iron supplements, or prescribed medication. The seeds replace valuable B vitamins, soothe the entire digestive tract, and have no known harmful chemical or drug interactions. Do not use, however, if you have diverticulosis, as the seeds may cause irritation.

CRAMPS AND SPASMS

Calcium. Frequent muscle spasms and cramping are often an indication of too little calcium in the diet. Drink teas rich in calcium such as dandelion, oat straw, raspberry, and plantain leaf. Common foods rich in calcium include almonds, carob, sesame seeds, yogurt, and most deep green vegetables.

Lavender. Lavender is both antispasmodic and sedative. Drink as a tea, or apply directly to the area as a wash or poultice for direct relief.

HOMEMADE CALCIUM SUPPLEMENT

Make your own daily calcium supplement by filling a jar halfway with organic crushed eggshells. Cover with vinegar and let sit for 2 weeks. Strain, then take 1 to 3 tablespoons daily. You can use this as salad dressing, in sauces, or sweetened with honey for a refreshing beverage, so you don't feel like it's medicine.

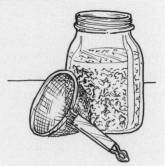

Mullein leaf. When smoked, mullein can instantly relax the bronchial spasms associated with asthma, whooping cough, and bronchitis.

Ginger. Drink ginger tea to relieve either stomach or menstrual cramping.

DETOXIFICATION

Dandelion and burdock root. If you buy an herbal detoxification formula, chances are its prime ingredients will be either dandelion or burdock root. But why buy it when you can get the fresh root for free? They are used worldwide whenever liver-related problems are involved. Both promote kidney function, too, and have abundant minerals to replace any that may be eliminated in urine. Dandelion tremendously benefits the digestive system, while burdock excels at alleviating chronic skin disorders and eruptions.

Red clover. Daily doses of red clover tea will help reduce the symptoms from steroids, radiation, or chemotherapy. It also has mild blood-thinning capabilities, making it useful as a preventative for arteriosclerosis and high cholesterol.

Thyme. Drink a cup of thyme tea to recover from a wild time. It will ease headache, nervousness, and the queasy stomach of a hangover more effectively and safely than over-the-counter sedatives or pain relievers.

Borage. Borage seed oil helps ease the stress from long-term chronic metabolic disorders such as menopausal distress, alcoholism, obesity, and steroid treatments. It also offers quick relief to a hangover.

DIARRHEA

Diarrhea can quickly become dangerous. If it lasts for more than four days (one day for small children) and is not getting better, if the person vomits everything he drinks or drinks nothing, if there is blood in the stools, or if the person is dehydrated and getting worse, prompt medical attention should be sought.

Rehydrating liquids. Any person with watery diarrhea is in danger of dehydration, especially a child. Do not wait until dehydration begins to start replacing lost fluids. Administer sips of a rehydrating drink every five minutes day and night until urination is normal. For babies, it is best to take the

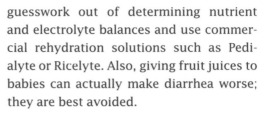
guesswork out of determining nutrient and electrolyte balances and use commercial rehydration solutions such as Pedialyte or Ricelyte. Also, giving fruit juices to babies can actually make diarrhea worse; they are best avoided.

Starchy fluids. These are a great cure for diarrhea. Make a thick oatmeal drink by cooking together 1 cup of oats and 2 quarts of water for 5 minutes. Strain and drink frequently in small sips. Starchy fluids tend to diminish vomiting and reduce fluid loss (unlike sweetened sugary drinks and sodas). If possible, make the drink with herbs that have high potassium content, such as alfalfa, borage, clover blossom, dandelion, raspberry, and pine needles.

Blackberry root. This has been the herb of choice to eliminate diarrhea and dysentery throughout history. Make the standard medicinal dose, and drink 1 teaspoon every five minutes until the diarrhea is under control. Repeat as necessary. Its milder cousins, raspberry and rose leaf, may be used in the form of a tea for small children.

Yogurt. This is one of the safest foods you can eat to prevent diarrhea because it is unlikely to have *E. coli* bacteria, the main cause of food poisoning. Eating plain yogurt daily also helps prevent diarrhea, as does drinking vinegar beverages sweetened with honey before meals.

Mullein. Mullein leaf tea is a mild astringent useful to help control diarrhea, especially in children. Add a tablespoon of plain yogurt to the mullein to offset its tannin content and add beneficial bacteria.

EARACHE

Olive oil and garlic. Plain olive oil is a traditional remedy used to soothe earaches quickly. Simply put a few drops of warm olive oil in the ear and have the person rest on their side with the ear up, for about five minutes so the oil has a chance to flow down into the inner ear. If agreeable to the patient, gently massage around the outside of the ear.

For further relief, I'll smash a clove of garlic and let it rest in warm olive oil for fifteen minutes and strain. Then, I'll take a one-inch cotton ball, let it soak up the garlic olive oil and place it so it rests just inside the outer earlobe. The cotton keeps the oil inside the ear, and the garlic helps combat the infection. Now have the patient turn and rest the troubled ear on a heating pad for about thirty minutes. The heat and gravity will help the ear drain, but the cotton will keep the oil from escaping. Repeat as needed, using fresh garlic and cotton each time. If the patient is prone to earaches, taking the above steps at the onset of colds or after swimming helps prevent ear infections in the first place — infinitely preferable to having to fight against an earache.

Always be sure the eardrum is not ruptured before putting anything in the ear. If the earache is persistent or recurring, consult a physician, as deafness may occur. Drink plenty of water, nutritive tonic herbs, and eat wholesome foods to build strength.

Mullein flower oil. Penelope Ody, a member of the National Institute of Medical Herbalists in the United Kingdom, cites in her book, *The Complete Medicinal Herbal,* the still-current use of mullein flower oil to soothe ear inflammations.

Plaintain. Drink plantain tea to help tone the delicate membranes of the inner ear. It also helps reduce chronic dizziness from ear inflammations.

Food allergies. Suspect food allergies if the ear infections are recurring. One study showed nearly 75 percent of a group of children scheduled to have tubes surgically placed into their ears showed sensitivity to milk, wheat, eggs, peanuts, or soy products. It may take the infections several months to clear up after the food culprit is removed from the diet.

ENERGY-BUILDING TONICS

Traditionally tonic herbs were taken after a steady winter diet of dried, salted, fatty foods. They help rejuvenate the body and bring energy levels up to the high demands placed on it through spring, summer, and harvest chores. Tonics nourish and promote general health of the internal organs, especially the liver, a main detoxifying organ of the body.

Spring tonics. These are usually made from spring's abundant green growth. Sometimes they consist of nothing more than plates of lightly steamed or salad greens such as dandelion greens, young garlic shoots, mallow leaves, and plantain or violet leaves and blossoms. Roots from dandelion or burdock that overwintered can be included for extra detoxifying action and to add depth to the flavor.

Winter tonic. Strawberry leaf tea is a simple old-fashioned wintertime tonic. Abundant in vitamin C, green year-round, strawberry also helps improve circulation to fight off winter's cold from within.

General tonics. Dandelion and burdock roots are two of the best general tonics that nature has to offer us. They may be combined or used separately; fresh, tinctured, or dried; in foods or as medicines; and some form of each is available year-round . . . whew, with flexibility like that no wonder these are so highly esteemed by herbalists around the world!

Blood tonic. Red clover blossom tea is a standard old-time blood tonic, and has often been used in conjunction with other herbs such as violet, burdock, dandelion, and garlic for the treatment of cancer and tumors. Today you'll see it frequently employed to help reduce the serious side effects from radiation and chemotherapy treatments.

MY ALL-AROUND NOURISHING TONIC

Nature has a capricious whimsy that can become a bit of a sore thorn when you start to gather your own plants for medicine. One year may be great for red clover, and then there may not be another good crop for four or five years. It's frustrating to learn an herb only to be unable to get enough the next year. So rather than rely on one herb, I make what I fondly call my backyard blend.

The blend changes from year to year depending on what nature has grown in abundance and what I've happened to gather. I simply dry the herbs, put them all together in one big paper bag, and grab a handful when I want a cup of nourishing tonic tea. The herbs are always nourishing simples such as red clover, borage leaf and flower, violet, plantain, alfalfa, and rose petal or hips. Unlike an herbal formula tailored to a specific ailment — where you try to keep the variety of herbs to a minimum — in this instance I use as wide a variety of simple foodlike herbs as possible, to get a broad spectrum of vitamins and minerals and to create a general nourishing tonic.

EYES

Rub your palms together briskly until they are quite warm. Now press your palms to your eyes for quick relief from eye strain, tiredness, and slight twitches.

Cool compresses. Soothe hot, inflamed eyes by placing cool compresses of plantain, lemon balm, or rose water on them. Let rest for five minutes at a time. This also can be used to clean away excessive eye mucus from conjunctivitis or pink eye.

Borage. Borage leaf was much valued by the ancient Greeks for strengthening weak eyes and preventing cataracts. Recent studies show you are eleven times more likely to develop cataracts if your diet lacks in beta-carotene, folic acid, and vitamin C. Borage has plenty, as do many other dark leafy greens such as dandelion and violet.

> ### SOOTHING BABY'S MINOR EYE IRRITATIONS
>
> Nursing mothers have the perfect remedy for baby's minor eye irritations and inflammations. Simply use a squirt of breast milk as a soothing wash. Breast milk is sterile as it leaves the breast, warm, and soothing; it also contains the mother's natural antibodies to help ward off infection.

FEVERS

Fever is the way the body kick-starts the immune system, and it may not be necessary to do anything but give the patient rest and plenty of fluids, and let nature take her course. Generally, this holds true if the fever stays under 100°F and lasts for no more than several days. Water is fever's nemesis. Flush the fever from the body by having the patient drink plenty of soothing and pleasant-tasting herb teas such as lemon balm, mallow-violet, rose hip, and lavender, or plain water.

Fruit teas. As a fever mounts, digestion slows. Avoid eating foods that are hard to digest. Instead drink mild, cooling fruit teas such as strawberry, raspberry vinegar, or rose petal tea.

Poplar bark. This should *not* be used to relieve fevers aches and pains in young children, as it contains the chemical precursor to aspirin and may cause complications. It may, however, be safely used by adults in combination with an emollient herb such as mallow or plantain.

> ### WARNING
>
> A fever that continues to rise or rises rapidly may be an indication of a systemic bacterial infection. Seek immediate medical treatment.

Borage. A cup of strong, warm borage lemonade will cool a fever while stimulating the kidneys to flush poisons from the system. The high vitamin and mineral content will help the person regain strength.

Encourage sweating. Burdock, catnip, ginger, and peppermint encourage sweating, and may be used as teas or baths to help break moderate fevers.

To bring down a fever, frequently sponge the patient's neck, forehead, ears, armpits, groin, and soles of feet with tepid brews of peppermint, catnip, or ginger. Have the patient drink as much water as possible, but in small frequent sips. Administer a teaspoon to a tablespoon of peppermint, catnip, or ginger tea every five minutes until the fever lowers.

FLU PREVENTION

The best prevention against viral infections is the resounding good health that comes from adding fresh herbs to your daily diet. Growing up in a medical family, and later working in a restaurant, I have been able to witness firsthand how easily germs are spread. Keeping your hands away from your eyes, nose, and mouth and washing them frequently will go a long way toward ensuring that the season's flu passes you by.

Garlic. Add 1 to 2 cloves of fresh raw garlic into your daily diet. Fresh garlic can be sprinkled on top of salads, soups, or bread, or mixed with honey, to minimize possible stomach upsets.

Thyme. This herb has potent antiviral and antibiotic qualities. Start drinking thyme as your daily beverage when everyone around you is getting the flu. If it is too late and you are already ill, thyme tea will lesson the duration and severity of the illness.

Rose hips. These are one of nature's best sources of vitamin C, and complement the flavor of nearly every herb you may choose to use to prevent colds and flus. Other herbs that are a good source of vitamins C or A are alfalfa, catnip, lemon balm, plantain, strawberry leaf, violet leaf, and white pine needle.

Violet. The common violet acts as a gentle immune-system stimulant. Drink a tea made from the whole aboveground portion of the plant. Other herbs that help stimulate the immune system to combat viral infections are St.-John's-wort, white pine, and strawberry leaf.

Yogurt. Plain yogurt can kill bacteria all on its own, but it will also help your body gear up for production of antibodies to kill invading organisms.

FROSTBITE

Mullein. Topical applications of mullein flower oil speed recovery from frostbite.

Mallow root. Make a warm mash of equal amounts of mallow root and oatmeal. Apply as a paste to the affected parts to help hold the heat to the area, and to soothe and protect.

Peppermint. Drink a tea made from equal amounts of peppermint and young strawberry leaf to help improve overall circulation.

Ginger. A salve made from peppermint or ginger can be applied before going out into cold conditions for long periods of time. The oil will protect the skin while the herb brings the blood to the area, thus helping to prevent frostbite. Small amounts of powdered ginger may also be simply sprinkled directly into your shoes.

Plenty of water. One of the secrets the most successful mountain climbers have is to drink copious amounts of water, because during extremely cold weather, the body loses a lot of moisture. If you know you'll be outside for an extended period of time, drink plenty of water, avoid consuming alcohol, and wear protective layered clothing.

GRAY HAIR

Folklore gives us many ways to prevent gray hair, and research lends credibility to some of the claims. Studies show that a diet lacking in any one of the following nutrients (they're all in the B vitamin group) produces lack of hair pigmentation, resulting in gray hair: folic acid, pantothenic acid, biotin, and para-amino-benzoic acid (PABA).

Unfortunately, the corresponding corollary that a diet rich in these nutrients reverses graying hair isn't quite accurate. Genetic tendencies and individual needs mean that what works for the goose doesn't always work for the gander. Folic acid seems to be the most effective nutrient in reversing gray hair. Biotin comes in a close second, but sometimes a combination of the two, or three, or even all four nutrients is needed. And some hair will remain gray no matter what nutrients are added to the diet. There is no doubt, however, that these nutrients play a strong role in determining the color and health of your hair.

Although the most concentrated doses of these nutrients are found in the organ meats, notably liver and kidneys, the plant world has good sources also.

Folic acid. The term *folic acid* is derived from the word *foliage.* It is abundant in most dark leafy greens. You will find it in the spinachlike herbs plantain, mallow, violet, dandelion, and alfalfa, and also in flavorful lemon balm, catnip, peppermint, and red clover. (The roots contain little folic acid.)

Plantain seeds are an excellent source of easily assimilated B vitamins, and I have met several people who swear they owe their abundant dark hair (and the fact that lice, ticks, and mosquitoes leave them alone) to sprinkling crushed plantain seeds on each meal.

Italians claim to look young with dandelion flower wine and green salads that contain solid levels of all four B vitamins.

Black walnut coloring. Meanwhile, to cover up the gray, make an infusion from the hulls of the black walnut, and dab it on the gray spots for a deep brown color that stays for about four to six weeks and lasts even through daily shampooing.

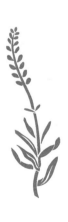

HEADACHE

Headaches (except for certain kinds of migraine headaches) are a symptom, not an illness in themselves. An estimated 90 percent of intermittent headaches stem from stress, eyestrain, colds and flus, dehydration, or fatigue. Once again, the classic remedy of rest and drinking plenty of fluids is bound to help. However, some headaches are due to inactivity. Simply step outside, breathe deeply, and go for a walk.

Calming teas. Drink calming and soothing teas such as catnip, lemon balm, lavender, rose petal, and violet. Or add them to a warm bath and let the water soak away your tension.

If the tension is concentrated in one area, apply hot compresses or a hot-water bottle to the area during the bath.

Rub the temples. Use an infusion or ointment made from lavender, peppermint, thyme, or ginger for tension headaches. Likewise, for sinus headaches, rub the sinus cavities with these warming herbs to help break up congestion.

Ginger. A daily drink of ginger has been shown to be nearly as effective at preventing migraines as powerful prescription drugs, with none of the debilitating side effects. Ginger oil can be rubbed onto the temples during early warning signs to thwart the oncoming migraine completely. To relieve pressure, soak your feet in a hot footbath with ginger or peppermint added to it. The bath draws the blood away from the head to the heat and provides a measure of relief.

Exhaustion. For headaches from nervous exhaustion, drink strong teas of alfalfa, St.-John's-wort, borage, or oat straw.

Poplar bark. An infusion of poplar bark will relieve most headaches in a manner similar to aspirin's. Combine with mallow root to ease possible stomach upset. (**Caution:** As with aspirin, poplar should *not* be taken by children with a high fever.)

> **WARNING**
>
> Chronic headaches may be an indication of severe problems. If the headache persists, bring it to the attention of a health professional.

HEART

Any heart trouble is potentially deadly serious and a health professional should be consulted at signs of trouble. However, simple herbs have a remarkable ability to keep trouble from arising in the first place.

Garlic. This remarkable plant is accepted as beneficial to the heart by both traditional and modern medicine. Garlic reduces cholesterol, reduces the buildup of fatty deposits in the arteries, lowers blood pressure, and helps prevent blood clots from forming — with no harmful side effects, and as effectively as some pharmaceutical drugs! Research shows that garlic may even prevent a second heart attack if you've had one already. The good news is that the compounds that give garlic its circulatory benefits are present in its every form: fresh, cooked, dried, and even powdered.

Use homemade preparations of garlic whenever possible. You will save tremendous amounts of money. Also, the main reason most people use capsules is to reduce the odor of garlic — but if the odor is missing, so are the many benefits of garlic.

Wine. If alcohol presents no problem to you, statistical evidence shows that drinking a glass of red wine before dinner will reduce the risk of heart attack by as much as 30 percent! Red wines seem to be slightly more beneficial than white. Home-made wines with herbs that enhance circulation, such as red clover, will add an extra benefit. However, even moderate alcohol consumption may bring on chest pain if you have angina, and those who drink more than a glass a day are putting themselves at risk for other health problems.

Oats. Three decades of research confirms the power of oatmeal to drive down cholesterol. All it takes is 2 ounces of oat bran a day, or ⅔ cup of oatmeal. Oats have a soluble gummy fiber that helps prevent cholesterol from being absorbed during digestion and thus keeps it from entering the bloodstream.

Walnuts. Even though walnuts are high in fat, it is a type of fat that helps lower cholesterol! In an otherwise low-fat diet, eating a few nuts a day (2 ounces) can help reduce cholesterol levels as much as 18 percent.

Vitamins and minerals. Eating fruits and vegetables rich in vitamin C, beta carotene, potassium, and vitamin E can help detoxify bad cholesterol and lower high blood pressure. Some of the twenty-five basic herbs used in this book (see pages 32–43) that are good sources are alfalfa, borage, catnip, dandelion, lemon balm, mallow leaves, peppermint, plantain, red clover, rose hips, strawberry, raspberry, violet, and white pine needle.

Red clover has a special compound called coumarin that helps thin the blood and prevent clotting. Combine with alfalfa to receive ample amounts of the vitamins and minerals that strengthen blood vessel walls.

HEMORRHOIDS

Hemorrhoids are varicose veins of the rectum. They may be painful but generally are not dangerous. They frequently appear during pregnancy, or may indicate poor nutrition. It helps to eat plenty of fruit, leafy greens, and foods with a lot of fiber (such as oats) to prevent constipation and rebuild the strength of the delicate membranes.

Astringent plant juices. Dabbing the juice of one of these plants on the hemorrhoids will help shrink them: blackberry leaf, poplar bark, raspberry leaf, or rose leaf or bark. These are all strong astringents.

Mullein. Mullein flower oil will help relieve pain and itching from external hemorrhoids.

INDIGESTION

Antacids are two of the top ten items purchased in grocery stores across America! TV commercials have convinced us that the cause of our indigestion is too much acid; actually, however, the average person has too *little* acid. A healthy person's stomach manufactures a strong acid called hydrochloric acid (HCL). As we become older, our diet deficient, or our life stressful, our body produces less and less HCL. Taking antacids often starts a vicious downspiral in which more and more are needed to prevent indigestion, while our food is actually not being digested at all! Symptoms of too little acid can be exactly the same as those of too much. Do not use antacid tablets until you have *confirmed* you really do have an overacid stomach.

Slow down and chew. We are always in such a hurry that we gulp through our meals, rush off to the next project, and complain when our stomachs rebel. Simply taking the time to enjoy your meal, chew your food, and savor the flavor is all the "medicine" it may take to eliminate indigestion altogether.

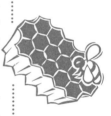

Sweetened vinegar. If you are lacking in stomach acid, the simplest way to add acid to your diet is with sweetened vinegar beverages. Simply put 1 tablespoon in a cup of water, sweeten with honey, and drink the tea ten to fifteen minutes before your meal.

Yogurt. Because of the high use of broad-spectrum antibiotics in this country, indigestion may be caused by a lack of beneficial intestinal bacteria. A sure remedy is to eat at least a cup of plain yogurt or other cultured milk such as kefir and acidophilus each day.

Mint. Few plants aid digestion in as pleasant a way as mint. Though we are familiar with mint in candies, ice creams, jams, and even cigarettes, these commercial products use mint extracts, which just cannot compete with the wonderful flavor and fragrance of fresh-picked green mint. Simply smelling fresh peppermint makes my mouth water and stirs up my appetite. Added to a salad (as is done throughout the Near East), it makes a wonderful meal starter that keeps indigestion from occurring at all. When the mint is blended with other greens, vegetables, and oil and vinegar, it does not overpower the salad as you may think, but instead simply adds a freshness to the whole spectrum of flavors.

Mint tea is a worldwide favorite remedy for upset stomach, nausea, flatulence, and weak appetite. It is safe enough for very small children — though they may prefer the milder flavor of spearmint.

Ginger. Ginger tea generally brings more warmth to stimulate digestion than does mint. The flavor is generally preferred by adults; also, strong ginger can cause unpleasant hiccupping and belching in small children. Sucking on a piece of candied ginger is an alternative. Ginger is especially beneficial after a heavy meal.

Catnip. Cold catnip tea can be drunk before meals to stimulate appetite, and warm catnip tea drunk after meals to prevent gas. Catnip makes a pleasantly refreshing beverage, and was the beverage of choice for much of Europe before the introduction of Oriental tea. A slice of lemon enhances its flavor perfectly. Catnip is excellent for calming a nervous stomach. Traditionally, teas made from red clover or catnip were drunk to soothe and heal irritated stomach ulcers.

Thyme. Thyme tea is a classic remedy for the stomach chills or upsets associated with colds and flus.

INFANT AILMENTS

Infants and babies are especially vulnerable to complications from both illness and treatment. Always choose the least amount of intervention necessary to alleviate any problem. When using herbs, remember that they are medicine. Choose extremely mild herbs, such as catnip, spearmint, and oat straw, and make the tea weak by diluting it. Use one part standard infusion to three parts water for babies over three months old.

In most cases when a baby is ill, breast-feeding should be encouraged to continue. Indeed, an ideal way to administer simple herb teas is to have the mother drink the tea and let the baby receive the medicine indirectly through the breast milk.

Colic. Weak catnip tea is the surest remedy for infantile colic. It quiets the nervous system and eases gastric distress. Either the nursing mother can drink the tea and the baby receive it through her milk, or a warm poultice of catnip can be laid on the baby's stomach, or an eyedropperful of the tea can be squirted directly into the baby's mouth. Frequent colic may indicate a food sensitivity — perhaps to cabbage or to cow's milk — which may occur even if the nursing mother is the one eating the allergy-causing foods.

Umbilical stump. Paint a newborn's umbilical stump with honey to prevent infection and help it dry up quickly.

Diaper rash and cradle cap. An infusion of violet, lavender, or plantain tea can be used as a wash for diaper rash or cradle cap.

INFLAMMATIONS AND INFECTIONS

Mallow. Apply poultices of mallow root or mallow leaf to draw out infections and soothe inflamed tissues. Apply the poultice as hot as is tolerable, and then add a hot-water bottle or hot cloth on top to keep it warm. Renew the materials as they cool. Continue this treatment until relief is felt. This remedy works equally well with plantain leaves.

When my husband awoke to a wound with ugly red streaks radiating from a throbbing armpit (indicating blood poisoning), the doctor was unable to see him for several hours. So I treated it as above, and within an hour the swelling had noticeably improved, the throbbing decreased. By the time of the appointment, the red streaks were hardly noticeable, so we canceled and kept up the treatment. By morning the wound itself was nearly healed.

Red clover. Red clover blossom tea will help in all manner of internal inflammations, as it aids the functioning of the lymphatic system. It is equally useful for skin swellings and inflammations, especially arthritic swellings, gout, and external ulcers.

Arthritis. To help prevent arthritis flare-ups, drink alfalfa tea daily.

Violet. Violet poultices will soothe inflamed skin sores and abscesses, as well as help to draw out stubborn infections.

REMOVING SPLINTERS

Paul Kenwaubekesie, who grew up fishing Lake Michigan for a living, taught me this trick to draw out stubborn splinters.

Heat pine pitch until it is warm but still tolerable to be put on the skin. Place the warm pitch on the splinter and let rest until it cools to about skin temperature. Peel off. Usually the splinter comes out on the first try, but you can repeat as needed. Paul used this method to get out stubborn fish spines and scales, just like his grandfather before him.

ITCHING

Vinegar. To relieve itching, try compresses of lukewarm diluted vinegar (¼ cup vinegar per quart of water). Herbal vinegars such as plantain, violet, rose, and lavender will add an extra measure of relief.

Oats. For itching over large areas of skin, put 1 cup of oats in a muslin bag, tie it shut, and toss the bag into a lukewarm bath. The bag can later be remoistened and rubbed over specific areas.

Plaintain. Poultices of plantain or marsh mallow give relief. Simply dip the leaf in warm water to soften it, then bind it to the area with a cloth. Replace when the leaf no longer feels cool.

The skin wash tincture on page 57 works well when itching is due to poison ivy, parasites, or fungal infections. For a simple remedy, try washing with walnut leaf infusion.

Chronic eczema and psoriasis. If the itching is due to a chronic condition such as eczema, topical applications may provide symptom relief but will not address the cause. The skin is a major eliminative organ. When constant eruptions occur on the skin we must look to aid the internal eliminative organs — the kidneys, plus the major detoxifying organ, the liver. Daily doses of infused borage oil are sometimes all that is needed to prevent psoriasis and eczema flare-ups. Adding dandelion to the diet and medicinal doses of dandelion tea will aid both liver and kidney function. Burdock root (used as food or medicine) is most effective for enhancing liver function.

For long-term treatment of acne, eczema, ectopic skin, or psoriasis, a daily tea of burdock root, red clover blossom, and violet leaf is especially helpful. First simmer the burdock root for 10 minutes, then remove from the heat and add the violet leaf and red clover blossom.

KIDNEY AND BLADDER FUNCTION

Yogurt. Eating a cup of yogurt daily to prevent yeast and bladder infections may sound like an old wives' tale, but it really works. The culture must be live to have any effect. For extra relief, add a cup of yogurt to a warm bath, or douche with a tablespoon of yogurt mixed in a quart of warm water.

Burdock and dandelion. Both of these herbs gently stimulate the kidneys to increase the flow of urine, yet have enough vitamins and minerals to replace any that may then be excreted in the urine. Thus they are generally considered safe for long-term use. Dandelion has a greater capacity for clearing obstructions from the kidneys and bladder, while burdock eases the strain on the kidneys by promoting sweat and encouraging the skin to eliminate toxins as well.

Bladder infections. These are the second most common complaint (next to menstrual difficulties) of women. Frequently they coincide with ovulation or pregnancy. Underwear traps bacteria and moisture and creates an ideal breeding ground. Wear none, or wear loose-fitting cotton underwear that breathes, if you are prone to infection. Also, drink copious amounts of water to dilute bacteria concentrations and increase urination; this helps the body rid itself of the bacteria. Avoid caffeine, as it irritates the kidneys; mild diuretics such as dandelion or burdock root help, though. Drinking ½ to 2 cups of cranberry or blueberry juice incapacitates the *E. coli* bacteria responsible for causing the infection. Drink ½ cup daily as a preventative or increase to 2 cups daily to help combat a current infection.

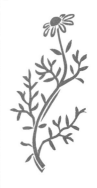

A tea made from equal parts of mallow root, dandelion root, and plantain leaf will relieve kidney and bladder infections. Plantain, especially, helps the kidneys secrete uric acid and is therefore helpful in attacks of gout.

Whenever administering an herb to increase the flow of urine, I add a demulcent herb such as mallow to help soothe any irritated tissue and to ease the possible passage of stones.

Sluggish kidneys. Compresses of warm ginger applied to the abdomen help stimulate sluggish kidneys, without necessarily increasing urine output.

Kidney stones. Drinking daily infusions of rose hip tea has been demonstrated to be useful in preventing and breaking up kidney stones.

MENSTRUATION AND PREGNANCY

It is no coincidence that a highly processed, high-fat diet lacking in fresh vitamins and minerals and menstrual difficulties go hand in hand. Although we have come to accept menstrual cramps, heavy or irregular bleeding, migraines, hot flashes, PMS, and mood swings as normal, they are indications that the body is not able to balance its hormonal cycle in a healthy manner. If you look carefully at most women's herb formulas, they are really nutritional supplements. Commonly used herbs such as dandelion, motherwort, raspberry leaf, burdock root, and nettle are powerhouses of easily assimilated vitamins and minerals.

Diet. Before addressing any symptoms of menstrual distress, look to your overall diet. Are you eating ample amounts of *fresh* fruits and vegetables? Are they organically grown? Do you eat store-bought meat and dairy products, most of which contain low-level amounts of antibiotics and hormonal supplements and so have a disruptive influence on your own hormonal cycle? Do you eat fresh whole grains? Every step you take toward eating good wholesome food is a step toward achieving a balanced cycle.

Borage. Borage seed oil will help the adrenals move stagnant energy in the body and relieve chronic menstrual difficulties such as PMS and difficult menopause. Sprinkle your food with alfalfa or plantain seeds or sprouts to add valuable B vitamins.

Strawberry. Drink strawberry leaf tea daily over a long period of time to regulate the menstrual cycle.

Ginger. Ginger tea and warm ginger poultices will ease menstrual cramping and nausea.

PREGNANCY TONIC

My favorite tonic to ensure a healthy pregnancy consists of equal parts of raspberry leaf, alfalfa leaf, lemon balm, and plantain leaf. I drank this daily when I was carrying my twins, who were born to term. One weighed 7 pounds, 10 ounces, the other 8 pounds, 6 ounces — 16 pounds of baby altogether!

When a friend's rabbits had infertility problems, I suggested she add some of this tea to their water, and her rabbits bred like — well, rabbits. Since then, several women who previously could not conceive or carry a baby to term have tried this tea blend, and are now proud mothers (though that is no actual proof the herbs were responsible). It is primarily a nutritive formula; the raspberry leaf helps strengthen the uterus, the lemon balm eases stress, and the plantain adds internal soothing.

Warming herbs. Other warming stimulant herbs such as peppermint, catnip, and thyme (it isn't called mother of thyme for nothing) can be tried. Also, supplement the diet with herbs high in calcium such as alfalfa, dandelion, and red clover.

Mentrual flow. To control excessive menstrual flow, drink strong teas of red raspberry leaf or red rose petal.

To promote delayed menstruation, a cup of lemon balm tea may be all that is needed to help the person relax and flow with her cycle. In China, ginger tea has been traditionally used to bring on menstruation. This has led to much controversy over the use of ginger in another traditional manner — to help control morning sickness when pregnant. However, studies are showing that ginger used in food or as beverage teas to help control morning sickness is not harmful to pregnancy.

PMS. Ease PMS irritability magically with a bowl of oatmeal! The complex carbohydrates found in oatmeal (and other whole grains) work nearly as well as Valium in calming PMS tension, and the nourishing action of oats calms the nervous system.

MOUTH, GUMS, AND TEETH

Gum tissue. To maintain healthy gums while brushing your teeth, use a homemade toothbrush fashioned from the twig of the walnut, poplar, or rose. This will help tighten your gum tissues, reduce any inflammation, and have a mild anti septic action. Simply sharpen one end of a pencil-length twig to use as a toothpick and chew on the fibers of the other end to use as a brush. Remove the thorns from the rose first by rubbing the twig lightly with a knife.

Use long rose or blackberry thorns as a field toothpick. Naturally grown thorns are sharper than toothpicks, they hold a point longer, and their curved shape makes them easier to use.

Mouthwash. The simplest mouthwash of all is a fresh, aromatic, antiseptic leaf chewed slowly. Lavender, lemon balm, peppermint, and thyme all excel as mouthwashes.

Tooth whitener. Rub your teeth with a fresh strawberry to whiten them. Diluted strawberry and peppermint tincture makes an excellent antiseptic mouthwash.

Teething. Babies may get relief by chewing on a piece of fresh catnip or peppermint, or the freshly crushed leaf can be rubbed over the area.

Abscess. To relieve an abscessed tooth, rub the area with a fresh garlic clove cut in half, and eat 1 to 2 fresh cloves of garlic daily.

Tooth decay. We all have heard the studies that link tooth decay to sweets. Less known, however, is that poor nutrition is also linked to tooth decay. A diet abundant in minerals gives you the building blocks necessary to maintain healthy, cavity-free teeth. Add liberal amounts of mineral-rich herbs such as alfalfa, burdock, dandelion, and violet to your diet to keep your smile free and easy.

Thrush infections. Chew fresh garlic and eat lots of yogurt to combat thrush infections.

Cold sores. These stem from a viral infection and tend to recur when a person is ill or under stress. The easiest remedy I know of is to keep the sore painted with pure honey until it is healed, and add a little powdered garlic or thyme to speed the healing along.

Mouth sores. Narrow sores at the corners of the mouth are another sign of poor nutrition. Treat them with an antiseptic wash of thyme or lavender and add fresh whole grains, fruits, and vegetables to the diet, while eliminating sweets.

Suck on a pastille made from equal amounts of finely chopped balsam poplar buds and powdered plantain leaf to heal stubborn mouth sores and ulcers. If the sore stems from a viral infection, add an equal amount of powdered lemon balm leaf when making the pastille.

NERVOUSNESS

Lavender. A few drops of infused lavender oil or a lavender infusion can be rubbed on the temples to dispel nervous tension. Drinking lavender infusion will enhance the action.

Catnip. If a person has the tendency to place nervous tension in the stomach, infusions of catnip tea will help calm and relax. If there is vomiting, apply a warm poultice of catnip directly onto the stomach.

Oats. Oats and oat straw tea are specifically nourishing to the nerves. Anyone who has difficulty dealing with stress or has chronic nervous tension should be encouraged to eat oats daily.

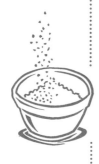

Lemon balm and rose petals. These both help lighten the heart and lift the spirits. Drink freely and as often as needed.

Poplar bark. To reduce pain from inflamed nerves, apply poultices of poplar bark, or St.-John's-wort oil, directly to the affected area.

Alfalfa. This makes a superlative tonic to speed recovery from nervous exhaustion or burnout, but has an aftertaste that many people do not enjoy. However, if you combine it with equal amounts of borage leaf and lemon balm, it makes a scrumptious lemonade-type beverage.

OVERWEIGHT

Chew well. "Fletcher" your food. In 1898 Horace Fletcher became the spokesperson for thoroughly chewing your food when he lost 60 pounds of fat in five months — with no other changes than chewing his food thoroughly, in a relaxed manner, and eating only when hungry. "Fletcherizing" became all the rage in his day, but studies still show that simply chewing your food to a pulpy liquid does indeed help with weight loss.

Ginger and spice. Eat spicy hot foods to rev up your metabolism and burn off fat. Drinking ginger tea may actually increase metabolism as much as 25 percent, helping you to burn off extra calories.

Digestion herbs. Herbs that aid digestion also help the body eliminate fat. Dandelion is the queen of the fat-burning herbs; mild in action, it will also replace any minerals lost to its slight diuretic action. Other herbs that help are burdock, catnip, lavender, and thyme.

For herbs to help combat fat in the blood (cholesterol and triglycerides), see the section on heart.

RECOVERY FROM LONG ILLNESS

The digestive system is most delicate immediately after illness. At first, thin oat broth may be all that can be tolerated. As the person grows stronger, try providing small amounts of well-cooked oatmeal; later, add crushed walnuts on top. Walnuts excel at rebuilding strength and promoting weight gain. Mild teas stimulate digestion — catnip, lemon balm, or dandelion — but at first, they may need to be weak infusions instead of standard strength.

Borage. Because of borage's unique building effect on the adrenal glands, it helps the body recover from stress and the lingering effects of steroid therapy, radiation, and chemotherapy. Borage seed oil, or borage leaf tea, is effective administered during and immediately after illness. As the person grows stronger, it is infinitely more fun to add fresh borage to the diet in salads, lemonades, syrups, or jams. Toss the salad with a walnut borage oil, and garnish with a few beautiful star-shaped blue borage flowers to please the eye as well as the palate.

Fresh greens. Long illness depletes the body of vital nutrients. Eat fresh greens and edible flowers to replace nutrients as efficiently as possible. Freely add alfalfa, burdock root, dandelion (flowers, greens, and roots), mallow (greens and cheeses), plantain (leaves and seeds), strawberry (leaves and blossoms), and violet (leaves and blossoms) into soups, salads, stir-fries, and desserts whenever possible, as well as strawberries, raspberries, blackberries, rose hips, and walnut meats.

Garlic. To help rebuild a weakened immune system, add 2 cloves of fresh garlic daily to the diet. Or, if the person's stomach cannot yet tolerate garlic, encourage a daily garlic footbath. Drink teas of thyme, St.-John's-wort, lemon balm, or violet to gently stimulate the immune system. St.-John's-wort and lemon balm have the additional benefit of easing the depression that invariably accompanies long-term illness.

SLEEP

Catnip, lemon balm, oat straw, and rose petal teas are all mildly sedative. Blend or leave as simples according to your personal tastes.

Bedwetting at night. This can be remedied by restricting water several hours before bedtime; also, have the person take a tablespoon of honey just before retiring. The honey will absorb excess moisture and eliminate the need for frequent bathroom trips.

Oversleeping. Needing too much sleep and lethargy may be signs of depression. St.-John's-wort has been shown more effective at relieving depression than commonly prescribed pharmaceuticals, with fewer side effects. Blend it with lemon balm and borage for greater effectiveness.

Conversely, if you need to stay awake, try a cup of strong ginger tea. Its stimulating warmth will invigorate your circulatory system to give a rush of energy without leaving any caffeine jitters behind.

Insomnia. Sleep on a pillow filled with dried lavender blossom, rose petal, and catnip to ease restlessness and insomnia. Children love to make these pillows, and it is a good way to introduce them to herbalism.

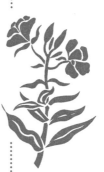

SMOKING TOBACCO (QUITTING)

Substitute herbs for tobacco. If you don't want to quit cold turkey, cut back on the amount of tobacco you use by adding herbs to it. Mullein leaf and a pinch of mint makes a fine smoke all by itself (or mullein leaf and rose petal, if you like a sweeter smoke). Each time you roll a cigarette, add more mullein and less tobacco. Most people can wean themselves from tobacco in a short time in this way.

Other herbs that make for a pleasant smoke are blackberry blossom, catnip leaf, lemon balm leaf, mullein flower, strawberry blossom, and violet flower. Old-timers used to smoke corn silk in their corncob pipes. It has a mild and pleasant taste that blends well with other herbs.

Chewing herbs. Chew on a piece of marsh mallow root or candied ginger, or on fresh rose hips.

Easing withdrawal. To ease the nervous anxiety that comes from nicotine withdrawal, use borage seed oil, and drink lemon balm or oat straw tea.

A double-blind placebo study has shown that extracts of fresh oats can reduce the craving for cigarettes. In the test, five out of the thirteen oat eaters stopped smoking, seven cut back by 50 percent, and only one person kept smoking as before. The effect lasted for as long as two months after the smokers stopped eating the oats!

Drink copious amounts of water to flush the nicotine from your body. Or take hot baths with ginger or peppermint added, to bring on a sweat, cleanse the toxin from your body, and help you relax.

SORE THROATS

Nibble on fresh young borage leaf, dried or fresh mallow root, a small piece of poplar bark, or violet blossom. Or, if you are brave enough, chew a piece of fresh raw garlic for fast relief.

White pine. A strong infusion of white pine needle tea will coat the throat with its antiseptic resins and provide generous amounts of vitamins A and C. Or suck on homemade thyme and balsam poplar bud pastilles.

Herbal syrup. A teaspoon of an herbal syrup will provide relief. Syrups made from borage, catnip, garlic, lavender, lemon balm, mallow, peppermint, plantain, poplar, red clover, rose, strawberry leaf, thyme, or white pine inner bark will aid a sore throat.

Gargle. Antiseptic gargles will help combat and prevent strep throat. Make a strong tea of thyme, peppermint, garlic, or white pine inner bark; gargle and swallow.

STRAINS AND SPRAINS

Use RICE to treat sprains and sprains. No, I don't mean the grain. RICE is an acronym for Rest, Ice, Compression, and Elevation. As soon as you suspect a sprain, keep the joint as motionless as possible, and elevate it over the person's head to relieve pain and swelling. Wrap it with an Ace bandage for firm support, and apply ice packs during the first twenty-four hours. Many times it's impossible to know if a hand or foot is bruised, sprained, or broken unless an X ray is taken.

Plaintain. Plantain leaf will cool an area and provide further relief from swelling and inflammation. Bind the bruised leaves directly onto the area, wrap loosely with a compression bandage, and apply ice on top. The plantain should be changed every other hour or so. Don't leave the plantain on overnight, as it can become lumpy if the person sleeps restlessly.

After twenty-four hours, use warm compresses and soaks of herbs that help reduce swelling, bruises, and inflammation. Borage leaf, plantain, poplar bark, and violet or walnut leaf will aid the recovery process.

Tea. Drink a blend of poplar bark and lemon balm tea to ease pain and inflammation, and to lift the spirits.

MAKING A COMPRESSION BANDAGE

In some emergency situations in which a hospital is not nearby, you may need to make a field cast or compression bandage. This can be made from white pine. Put 1 pound of white pine branches, with their needles, into 1 gallon of water and boil until it is reduced by half. Strain and boil until a thin syrup forms. Dip strips of flannel or muslin into the syrup.

Now use as follows: Make sure the sprained joint is in a good position. Wrap the joint in a soft clean cloth, then follow with a layer of cotton, cattail down, or other soft filling. Finally, put on the wet cloth strips so that they form a firm but not overly tight bandage. Do **not** put the strips directly against the skin. Made properly, this bandage will lend enough support to enable the person to walk out of the wilderness with the aid of a walking stick.

WARTS

Saliva. The most convenient remedy I know of for warts is simply to rub your own saliva on them several times a day. The enzymes in your saliva that help break down the protein in your food also help break down the structure of the wart. This works very well for children, who may have a sea of warts clustered in an area. Of course, it helps to give the child a special magic chant to say when he spits on the wart. "I wish, I wish, I wish, the warts would go away." Magic and superstition, yes . . . but it always helps to believe in what you do.

Dandelion. Apply the white sap from the stem or root of dandelion directly to the wart at least once a day. It is just corrosive enough to be effective against the wart, but it leaves the surrounding tissue undamaged.

Rose hip seed oil. The high vitamin E content of rose hip seed oil will help soften stubborn plantar warts. Then dandelion juice can be applied to dissolve them away.

There are many anecdotal stories of stubborn and persistent warts disappearing when a person turns from a high-protein (meat-based) to a high-carbohydrate (vegetarian) diet.

WORMS, PARASITES, AND FUNGAL INFECTIONS

Most home remedies to expel worms and parasites incorporate modified food fasts. Eating only raw cabbage or carrots is considered a remedy by itself — but I sure can't get my children to stick to that for the three to five days required! A more successful approach is to lean the diet toward eating lots of beans, rice, cabbage, and carrots for about a week while drinking lots of water and demulcent teas (such as borage or plantain leaf), trying the herbal therapies below, and taking any side indulgences with a grain of salt.

Garlic. Garlic is superior to many prescription drugs at eliminating parasites because it often works just as fast but is much safer and less expensive to use. Garlic can wipe out *Giardia lamblia* in as little as three days, and pinworms overnight! Chop a clove of fresh garlic and take with each meal, along with one additional dose of garlic before retiring. Fresh garlic works fast and efficiently; garlic oils, capsules, and powders do not. A wash with garlic wine or garlic water as made on page 108 will quickly eliminate ringworm, athlete's foot, and other fungal infections. Since garlic's parasite-fighting qualitites are destroyed by heat, follow instructions for making simple tea from leaves and flowers on page 29. For best results, continue using the garlic until the egg-laying cycle of the parasite has passed.

Walnuts. Walnut hulls and bark expel intestinal worms and parasites from the body. They are especially useful for skin-related parasites and may be safely used both externally and internally. The one drawback is that a wash made with the hulls will stain the skin a patchy dark brown that lasts for several weeks — about as long as a Florida tan! However, since their action is sure and mild, walnuts are often employed by those who may disdain garlic for one reason or another.

Thyme. Eating sprigs of thyme in salads or sandwiches, or drinking thyme tea, is an old English remedy to expel round-worms and pinworms.

Urine. Use your own urine to cure stubborn cases of athlete's foot! The urine creates an environment that the athlete's foot fungus cannot tolerate, plus it actually soothes the inflammation and itching. Just spread your toes wide to get between the cracks, let them air-dry, and go barefoot as much as possible. Also consider trying a urine bath. Use one cup urine to one gallon water and soak your feet for about fifteen minutes, or employ it as a spongebath to combat fungal infections spread over other areas of the body.

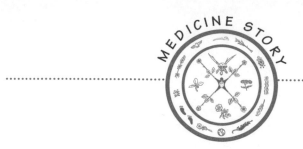

GOOD MEDICINE

Odemin had great power when he was a medicine man, but his power became greater after he became a strawberry. Once, first man and first woman were having a fight, and the woman had enough and fled from the man. When the woman didn't return the next day, the man tried to go after her, but he couldn't catch up. So he asked for help.

Creator took pity on man and flung raspberries in the path of the woman to slow her down, but the woman's anger was so great that she let the thorns tear at her as she raced through the tangle. Next Creator tried blackberries, then roses, then every other fruit he could think of, but nothing slowed her down.

Finally Odemin, the strawberry, lay down before her feet. She was so captivated by the beauty of this plant that she stopped to look. When she tasted a fruit it was so delicious she just had to have another. But the berries were so tiny it took her hours to gather a handful. This gave first man a chance to catch up with her and mend their quarrel.

It is said that when a person with a good heart dies, he will see a tremendous strawberry on his path as his spirit walks west. He can easily grab handfuls of this strawberry and it will nourish his soul for the journey ahead. But if his heart was small and bitter, there may not be enough strawberry for him to finish his journey. Then he must wait for another person to come along who has a strawberry big enough to carry the two of them.

Just as the strawberry is connected to the plant by a vast system of runners, leaves, and roots, so too is your heart connected to all the organs of your body, and your soul to all the parts of your family, your community, the planet, and the universe. We are constantly sending out new runners to explore new parts of our selves and the world. Thus strawberry reminds us that for healing to be complete it must take place in a physical sense, as well as a spiritual one. It represents the beginning, because it is the first berry to ripen. It also represents the end, because its spirit is with us at our physical end. It can represent the duality of all things and the cycles of the universe. Always look to the nature of a plant. Every plant tells a different story.

CONCLUSION
The Spirit of Herbalism

*The roots of a plant go down, and the deeper they go
the more moisture they find.*

— Okute, *Teton Sioux*

I started this book saying that healing begins the moment we decide to heal ourselves. When we heal ourselves with plants we have gathered, we have begun to heal our spirit as well as our body. We send out invisible runners that help us put into perspective our place in nature, and on some level we also make a connection with the spirit of the plants. Enough studies have been done to demonstrate clearly the beneficial effects that gardening or simply being in a garden has on mentally ill, depressed, and criminal behaviors. Not as well documented are the effects of plants on normal behavior. But think for a moment: How do you feel after you water your lawn or garden? Why do most of us have houseplants? Certainly not because we need one more thing to keep us busy! There can be no denying that plants speak to us on some level — they just don't use a language that can be put into words.

DEVELOPING OUR SEVENTH SENSE

Imagine for a moment you are packing for a trip. Into your suitcase you put your shirts, socks, an extra pair of pants, a book to read on the airplane, tickets, money, a jacket, a hairbrush, soap, Aunt Martha's present . . . and what else? What did you forget? As you drive to the airport the feeling that you've forgotten something grows and grows. You get on the plane, take off, and are in midair when all of a sudden you remember you forgot . . . your toothbrush! Now you can finally relax. It doesn't even matter that you can't go back and get your toothbrush. That nagging feeling of forgetting something was your subconscious's way of screaming at you — only it doesn't know words. So it kept at you, until the moment when you stopped thinking about it and all of a sudden the answer came — Oh, yes, my toothbrush! Remember that tightness and release when you go to learn from the plants themselves. They don't speak in words, either.

Learning to listen to your subconscious voice is an indispensable tool when you work with the plants. How do you know whether to gather the plant on your right, the one on your left, or the one in the middle? How do you know to gather today or tomorrow? Certainly you can learn the rational reasons, but on some level you also must learn to get a feel for the plants.

This is where herbalism and pharmacology split. Pharmacology demands that we know the exact amount of the medicinally active ingredient we are using; such a measurable dose is necessary for treatment and studies. Herbalists recognize that dosage is largely a question of experience. It is rarely possible to calculate the proper dose of an herb preparation without special equipment and testing. However, as many herbs are only weakly active and essentially nontoxic, the therapeutic amount prescribed is large and the question of dose is of minor significance.

Exercises for Learning to Listen to the Plants

Here are several fun exercises for you to try — by yourself or with a friend — to help you gain experience and learn to trust yourself with plants beyond rational thought.

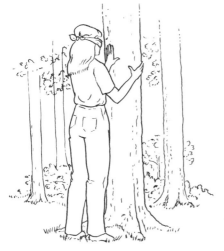

BLINDFOLD HIDE AND SEEK
Have a friend blindfold you and walk you some distance to a grove of trees. Have her lead you to a particular tree and let you spend about twenty minutes or so exploring that one tree — in whatever way feels best to you. With the blindfold still on, have your friend lead you back to your starting point. Take your blindfold off and go see if you can find your tree. It may take a while, but most people find their tree in less than half an hour. Still doubt? Reverse the process and blindfold your friend.

VALIDATE YOURSELF

Pick a plant that intrigues you. Make yourself comfortable. Quiet your inner voice and run your hands up and down the plant. Place your hands on the ground where the plant's roots would be also. Now try to feel where the greatest concentration of energy is in the plant at that moment. If you feel like asking questions, be sure they are simple questions with yes or no answers. Remember 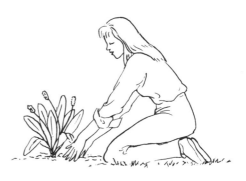 how you felt when you forgot the toothbrush — that is your individual subconscious negative response. How you felt when you remembered the toothbrush is your positive response.

At first most of us doubt the validity of any responses we have. Perhaps you keep thinking of the color red, and wonder what that has to do with anything. But each person brings his own previous set of experiences with him to this exercise. Colors, feelings, smells, sensations — each person will need to learn to decipher what these associations means to him personally. For most people it takes several attempts to decipher the subconscious code. The plants are patient; they will be there if you want to try again. What is most important is to know that on some level what you experience (or don't) is both real and valid.

GUESS WHICH HAND

Have a friend find two similar twigs that could be hidden in a hand — one alive and one dead. Take several minutes to calm and center yourself. Then, while your eyes are closed, have the friend place one twig in each one of your hands. Without looking, try to guess which twig is alive. I find about a 75 percent successful guess rate in small groups and workshops. But if you get into larger groups, or stressful or unfamiliar surroundings, this accuracy diminishes.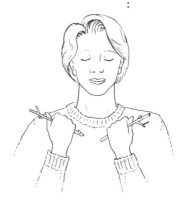

HEALING IS BALANCE

The preceding exercises help you key into developing your own connection with plants and medicine. The more you develop this connection, the more you will get the feel of when to add a pinch more or less of an herb to a brew or blend, which plant to pick and when. You will also bring the healing into your spirit as well as your body, and bring the two into balance.

Balance as a chronic state evokes health. At its best, our food becomes our medicine. Whole fresh foods become part of daily living, thereby preventing our tendency to move from one extreme to another. Every school of herbal medicine, from ancient Greek to modern Western, studies the relationship between the individual and the entire universe — and the resulting struggle for balance between the two.

How to Promote Balance

Many things promote balance: music, ritual, movement meditations, and, of course, plants. Some plants are balanced in themselves, but most have properties that bring us away from excess and back to balance. Perhaps this is why I am such an advocate of growing or gathering your own herbs. The very act is healing. It involves purpose, action, watching nature, and moving within her time frame, and it is always instructive. You gather an understanding of a plant's qualities in a way that never comes from merely opening a box or a bag. People who grow or gather are more likely to use the plant, because they intimately know how it feels and smells. Gathering demands that we create a personal relationship with the entire universe to achieve our balance with it.

> To forget how to dig the earth
> and tend the soil
> is to forget ourselves
> — Mahatma Gandhi

This is why the best herbs are not necessarily the strongest. Goldenseal, cascara bark, bearberry, and black cohosh are too strong to be used regularly. They are not moderate; they should be used only for extreme conditions when the body needs a jump-start toward health. The best herbs show no other effect than continuous good health. Often they cross over into being our foods: apple, barley, clover, dandelion, lamb's-quarter, mint, nettle, onion, strawberry, and thousands of others. These are the simplest herbs to use, understand, and gather. Ultimately, balance must be simple — or it misses its own definition.

THE NATIVE HEALING WHEEL: A GUIDE TO BALANCING THE ELEMENTS

Whichever path of herbalism you choose to follow — be it traditional Chinese or modern Western herbalism — your ultimate goal will be balance. How balance is sought is the key difference among healing systems. Modern medicine seeks balance by examining separate elements and then piecing them back together to form a whole picture. Traditional Chinese medicine draws on five thousand years of detailed observation and experience. There is a great deal of information available on these healing systems.

There is not as much discernible information on Native healing systems — perhaps because in them, healing lies within the individual. There is no one way to codify or key the person into a preexisting system . . . the person *is* the system. The only real rule is that healing must follow the Great Law of Peace — which is simply an agreement to get along with all of creation. Until each individual finds his own path, healing cannot begin for him.

Each person therefore takes responsibility for his own healing. A person's role in healing can be represented by a medicine wheel. The wheel is commonly employed to represent the circle of life, an idea, a vision, or a healing. Because the individual is at the center of the wheel, there can never be only one representative healing wheel. Each person brings his own interpretation of the universe to the wheel.

With this in mind, I have shaped a wheel representative of some of the considerations bought into play for healing in the Native American tradition. Plants, animals, and elements often change, depending on the person's age, well-being, clan and personal needs. What is most important is the balance among elements, not elements themselves.

Understanding the Wheel

Briefly, there are four directions on the wheel. This wheel represents only one plane in what is actually a sphere; keep in mind that an equally negative sphere exists, too. This other sphere could be viewed as the air between the spokes of a wheel. Together, the wheel is stronger than if it were one solid piece.

East. The east, where the sun rises, represents new beginnings. Its healing aspect is the mind, where the decisions of when and how to heal are made. Tobacco is most commonly its plant manifestation, since tobacco is customarily placed as an offering before embarking on a course or path.

South. The healing gift of the south is growth, or being in the present moment. Its aspect is the body and emotions, which intertwine and affect each other constantly. Cedar most commonly represents the south, because it keeps growing even when fallen and uprooted.

West. West is spirit energy, looking within for healing and death. It acknowledges that for healing to happen, transformation is necessary. Here is found the cleansing energy from burning or smudging with sage.

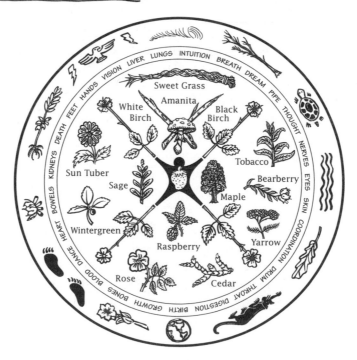

North. The north brings us wisdom, and the patience of winter and dormancy. The healing gifts of sleep, dreams, and vision lie in the north. Wisdom eases our mind and helps us think sweet thoughts, just as sweet grass does.

Center. Each person has his own center. The heart, represented by the strawberry, stretches out to the universe with a vast system of runners, leaves, and roots.

The whole. All these energies, along with those of nature and spirit, must be considered together for the work of healing to be complete.

Restoring Balance

A person may initiate and conduct his own healing. Fasting, sweat lodges, and vision seeking may be used to help restore balance. However, imbalance may have its roots in the person's family or community as well, or the person may simply need the support of others. So it is more common for healing to involve more than just the individual. This understanding is finally coming to modern medicine, which now recognizes that a person heals faster at home, surrounded by loved ones, than in an isolated and unfamiliar hospital setting. Americans may complain that home health care is only a way for the medical establishment to save dollars, but it also saves our sanity.

Using the Wheel:
The Universal Center and Ojibway Tea

Ojibway tea is a formula that was given to a Canadian nurse named Rene Caisse by an Ojibway medicine man (whose name seems lost to obscurity) as a cure for her mother's cancer. It is also called Essiac, which is *Caisse* spelled backward. The standard four-herb recipe is:

1   ounce sifted turkey rhubarb root powder (*Rheum palmatum*)
½   cup cut burdock root (*Arctium lappa*)
4   ounces slippery elm bark (*Ulmus rubra*)
16 ounces sheep sorrel herb (*Rumex acetosella*)

The medicine man was probably a member of the Mide (the Grand Medicine Society). Perhaps he envisioned the formula; perhaps it had been passed on for generations. Whichever the case, it is a remarkable example of how the wheel may be used to create an herbal formula. The blend is made of four herbs, and four is the number of balance on the wheel. Notice how the formula's components visually increase in increments of four. We have roughly 1 part (by volume) of rhubarb root to 4 times that amount of burdock and slippery elm, to 4 times that amount of sheep sorrel.

Burdock and rhubarb root would be placed in the west, as they are gathered in the fall and their medicinal qualities follow the body's deep internal rhythms. Slippery elm would be associated with the north simply because bark is one of the few things that can be gathered during the long frozen winters of the Far North. Also, the medicinal action of slippery elm affects the breath (spirit). Gathered in midspring and healing to the skin, sheep sorrel leaves bring the aspect of the east to the formula.

What is missing from this formula? A plant aspect from the south. Why? Because cancer is an imbalance of excessive growth, and the energy from the south is growth. Not only physical growth, but also the emotional, mental and visionary excesses of growth. To add herbs from the south (as some formulas add red clover blossoms) renders it less effective on a metaphysical level, according to the cosmology of the wheel.

The ultimate beauty of Native American herbalism is that it allows for your own personal preferences and differences. I have been told endless times when I ask about an herb, "Well, this is what worked for me, but I don't know if that will help you any at all." And if it is another theory of healing that you choose to follow, follow it well, because that is what works for you.

Accepting our innate differences is an intrinsic part of healing. Medicine is and always will be an art as well as a science. The best we can do is to follow the Great Law of Peace and agree that if we can't agree on anything else, at least we can agree to get along with one another.

THE CHALLENGE OF HERBALISM:
TOO MUCH TO LEARN

The *Wall Street Journal* now backs information as being more valuable than gold. The Internet has only increased our fear of being out of date. Every day there is so much more new information that we are hard pressed to keep up — it is the new stress for the new millennium. Indeed, the field of herbalism is a prime example. No one — even with a computer — can keep up with all the new information concerning plants and their medicinal attributes that is constantly developing or being bought to the forefront from modern research, the Amazon rain forests, the Ivory coast, ayurvedic medicine, Tibetan medicine, traditional Chinese medicine, and other means.

Great gobs of money is being spent trying to find patentable medicines and extracts to cure cancer, AIDS, leukemia, and even baldness — anything that people will spend great gobs of money to fix. In the past years I've seen feverfew change from a largely forgotten herb to one in the highest demand. Other fads will come and go: blue-green algae, wheat grass, *kombu-cha,* raw foods, and bee pollen, to name a few.

But the simple medicinal weeds in your backyard will always be there for you to use, without any multilevel marketing schemes, exorbitant price tags, dangerous side effects, exploitation of third-world child labor, expensive equipment, capital, or even fancy packaging to throw away. What do you think the people of post–World War II Germany turned to for medicine — encapsulated supplemental formulas, expensive Western pharmaceuticals, or tree bark? To this day Germany's reliance on herbal medicine sets the standard for the world. They learned firsthand to treasure their weeds. We can do the same.

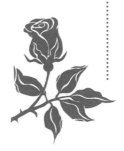

METRIC CONVERSION

Use the following formulas for converting U.S. Measurements to metric. Since the conversions are not exact, it's important to convert the measurements for all of the ingredients to maintain the same proportions as in the original recipe.

Measurement	Multiply by	to Convert to
teaspoons	4.93	milliliters
tablespoons	14.79	milliliters
fluid ounces	29.57	milliliters
cups	236.59	milliliters
cups	0.236	liters
pints	473.18	milliliters
pints	0.473	liters
quarts	946.36	milliliters
quarts	0.946	liters
gallons	3.785	liters
ounces	28.35	grams
pounds	0.454	kilograms
inches	2.54	centimeters
degrees Fahrenheit	$\frac{5}{9}$ (temperature − 32)	degree Celsius (Centigrade)

HOME REMEDY LIBRARY

Comprehensive Home Health Guides
Alternative Medicine, The Definitive Guide, compiled by the Burton Goldberg Group, Future Medical Publishing, Inc., 1995. Authoritative text from 380 leading alternative practitioners.
Columbia University College of Physicians & Surgeons Complete Home Medical Guide, Crown Publishing, 1995.
The Mayo Clinic Family Health Book, David E. Larson, M.D., Editor-in-Chief, William Morrow & Company, 1990.
Women's Bodies, Women's Wisdom, by Christiane Northrup, M.D., Bantam Books, 1994. Holistic approach to women's health concerns.

Field Guides
The Ecoherbalist's Fieldbook, by Gregory Tilford, Mountain Weed Publishing, HC 33, Box 17, Conner, MT 59827, 1993. Excellent for beginning gatherers; teaches not only what to gather, but also how.
Edible and Medicinal Plants of the Great Lakes, by Thomas Nagel, Wilderness Adventure Press, 1996. Thorough discussion of plants and uses with easy field identification guide.
Native Harvests, by Barrie Kavasch, Vintage Books, 1979. Includes recipes for everything from soups to nut cakes.
Newcomb's Wildflower Guide, by Lawrence Newcomb, Little, Brown and Company, 1977. Simple, effective key system for quick identification.

Peterson's Field Guide to Wild Edibles, Lee Allen Peterson, Houghton Mifflin Company, 1977.

The Peterson Series of Field Guides, Houghton Mifflin Company. The standard in field guides.

Stalking the Wild Asparagus, by Euell Gibbons, David McKay and Company, 1971. Factual, fun to read, and incredibly practical.

Herbal Reference Books

The Complete Illustrated Holistic Herbal, by David Hoffman, Element Books, 1996. References 200 herb applications, constituents, actions, preparations, and dosages.

The Complete Medicinal Herbal, by Penelope Ody, Dorling Kindersley Publishing, 1993. One hundred twenty common medicinal herbs and their applications.

Medicinal Plants of the Pacific West, by Michael Moore, Red Crane Books, 1993. One of the best books available on herbal medicine.

A Modern Herbal, by Maude Grieve, Dover Publications. Reprinted since 1931, one of the definitive sources on herbal medicine today.

The Way of Herbs, by Michael Tierra, Simon and Schuster, 1990. A blend of Eastern and Western herbal traditions in this classic.

Essential Oils References

The Complete Book of Essential Oils and Aromatherapy, by Valerie Ann Wormwood, New World Library, 1991. Excellent resource.

The Essential Oils Book, by Colleen K. Dodt, Storey Publishing, 1997. Presents a solid background in using essential oils.

The Healing Power of Aromatherapy, by Dr. Hasnain Walji, Prima Publishing, 1996. General and detailed information.

Nurse's Operative Manuals

These *optional* books are tools of the professional medical trade. They can help you determine when to seek a physician; show you how to safely care for a patient, provide long-term care, and handle an emergency; help you understand the nature of an illness; and provide valuable insights whatever course of treatment you pursue.

The Lippincott Manual of Nursing Practice, edited Sandra M. Nettina, Lippincott-Ravein Publishers, 1996. The standard nursing reference.

The Merck Manual of Diagnosis and Therapy: General Medicine, edited by Berkow & Fletcher, Merck & Company, 1992.

Other Recommended Herbals and Books

American Indian Medicine, by Virgil Vogel, University of Oklahoma Press, 1977. One of the most comprehensive writings on Native American theories of illness and methods of healing.

American Materia Medica: Therapeutics and Pharmacognosy, edited by Finely Ellinwood, Eclectic Medical Publications, 1983. An herbal medical pharmacopeia.

Botanical Influences on Illness, by Werbach and Murray, Third Line Press, 1994. A sourcebook of clinical research on herbal treatments.

The Crooked Tree, by John C. Wright, Matthew Erwin, publisher, 1917. Stories and legends of northwestern Lower Michigan.

Diet for the Atomic Age, by Sara Shannon, Avery Publishing Group, 1987. References the effect of diet on building and maintaining health, especially as concerning low- and high-level radiation.

An Elder's Herbal: Natural Techniques for Promoting Health and Vitality, by David Hoffman, Healing Arts Press, 1993. Gaia concept of healing.

Food — Your Miracle Medicine, by Jean Carper, HarperCollins Publishers, 1993. How your food affects your health.

The Green Kitchen Handbook: Practical Advice, References and Sources for Transforming the Center of Your Home into a Healthy Livable Place, by Annie Berthold-Bond, Mothers and Others for a Livable Planet, and Meryl Streep, Harper Collins, 1997. A practical how-to manual on how to make and maintain an organic kitchen inexpensively.

Growing and Using the Healing Herbs, by Gaea and Shandor Weiss, Wing Books, 1992. Information on growing medicinal herbs for home use.

Healing Power of Garlic, by Paul Bergner, Prima Publishing, 1996. Everything you needed to know about garlic, but never knew to ask.

Herbal Drugs and Phytopharmaceuticals, by Norman Grainger Bisset, CRC Press, 1994. Herbal drugs common in pharmaceutical practice — their constituents, indications, doses, and authentications.

Herbal Healing for Women, by Rosemary Gladstar, Fireside Books, 1993. A complete and holistic herbal health care manual for women.

Herbal Medicine, by Dian Dincin Buchman, Grammercy Publishing, 1979. An excellent general-purpose home herbal.

History of the Ottawa and Chippewa Indians of Michigan: A Grammar of the Language and Personal Family History of the Author, by Andrew J. Jackson (Chief Mack-aw-de-be-nessy), reprinted through the Little Traverse Regional Historical Society, Petoskey, MI, 1977.

How Indians Use Wild Plants for Food, Medicine & Crafts, by Frances Densmore, Dover Publications, 1974. An ethnological account of how the Ojibway of Minnesota and Wisconsin use their natural plant resources.

Indian Herbology of North America, by Alma R. Hutchens, Merco Publishing, 1973. How to use and prepare two hundred North American herbs.

Legends of Green Sky Hill, by Louise J. Walker, Wm. B. Eerdmans Publishing, 1977. Ojibway tales and legends.

Mishomas Book, The Voice of the Ojibway, by Edward Benton-Banai, Indian Country Press, 292 Walnut, Irvine Park Offices, Saint Paul, MN 55102, 1979. *Mishomas* is the Ojibway word for "grandfather." This book presents the teachings, prophecies, and insights of the Ojibway culture.

Nanaboozhoo, Giver of Life, by Alethea K. Helbig, Green Oaks Press, 1987. A compilation of oral and written history, legend and lore of Nanaboozhoo.

Nature Doctor, by Dr. H. C. Vogel, Instant Improvement Publishing, 1994. Recounts 65 years practicing natural and herbal medicine.

Nutrition and Degenerative Disease, by Weston Price, Keats Publishing, 1990. Analysis of the effects of primitive diet versus those of modern Western diet on degenerative disease. Excellent reading.

Nutritional Herbology, by Mark Pederson, Wendell Whitman Company, 1994. Nutritional profiles of most medicinal and culinary herbs.

Stalking the Healthful Herbs, by Euell Gibbons, Alan Hood, 1966. Practical applications and uses of common plants for home remedies.

RESOURCES

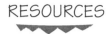

BOTTLES AND JARS
Honestly, the best source may be your local recycling center or resale shop. But if you want a particular jar, try one of these sources:

E. D. Luce Prescription Packaging
562-802-0515
www.essentialsupplies.com
Wholesale bottles, vials, jars, measuring, and apothecary supplies — by the case.

SKS Bottle and Packaging, Inc.
518-880-6980   Ext. 1
www.sks-bottle.com
Plastic, glass, and metal containers of all sizes and shapes at wholesale prices! I love their selection of blue glass and small lip balm containers.

Sunburst Bottle Company
916-929-4500
www.sunburstbottle.com
Wholesale priced. Beautiful and practical bottles.

SEED AND GARDEN SUPPLIERS

Abundant Life Seeds
541-767-9606
www.abundantlifeseeds.com
Organic open-pollinated heirloom seeds, and great book selection.

Bountiful Gardens
707-459-6410
www.bountifulgardens.org
Organic seeds, garden supplies, and educational projects.

Companion Plants
740-592-4643
www.companionplants.com
Certified organic medicinal herb plants.

Elixir Farm Botanicals
417-261-2393
www.elixirfarm.com
Chinese and indigenous medicinal organic plant seeds and nursery plants.

Gardens Alive! Inc.
513-354-1482
www.gardensalive.com
Organic pest controls and plant foods.

Johnny's Selected Seeds
877-564-6697
www.johnnyseeds.com
Medicinal herbs — some organic. Trial gardens open to public.

Native Seeds/ SEARCH
866-622-5561
www.nativeseeds.org
Traditional native American seeds for food and medicine.

Nichols Garden Nursery
800-422-3985
www.nicholsgardennursery.com
Herb and heirloom varieties.

North Country Organics
802-222-4277
www.norganics.com
Natural fertilizers, soil amendments, and natural pest controls.

Renaissance Acres Organic Herb Farm
http://raorganicherbfarm.com
Organic herb plants and seeds

Richters
905-640-6677
www.richters.com
Medicinal herb seeds.

Seeds of Change
888-762-7333
www.seedsofchange.com
Organic seeds.

Seeds Trust/High Altitude Gardens
928-649-3315
www.seedstrust.com
Seeds that are vigorous and tolerant of a harsh climate.

HERB AND NATURAL PRODUCT SUPPLIERS
If you cannot gather or grow your own herbs, try to support your local herb growers as much as possible. There are, however, some excellent herbalist-owned companies that sell their products through the mail.

Avena Botanicals
866-282-8362
www.avenaherbs.com
High-quality simple extracts, compounds, glycerites, oils, and blends for animals and people. Reading their catalog is a course in herbal medicine in itself.

Dry Creek Herb Farm
888-489-8454
www.drycreekherbfarm.com
An extensive listing of bulk organically grown and ethically wild-crafted herbs, along with a delightful line of skin care products, scents, and soaps.

From Nature with Love
800-520-2060
www.fromnaturewithlove.com

Jean's Greens
518-479-0471
www.jeansgreens.com
An excellent source of quality herbs.

Liberty Natural Products
800-289-8427
www.libertynatural.com
Herbal extracts, essential oils, and natural products.

Motherlove Herbal Company
970-493-2892
www.motherlove.com
Quality-certified organic and ethically wild-crafted herbs and products.

Mountain Rose Herbs
800-879-3337
www.mountainroseherbs.com
A small company carrying tools, equipment, bulk dried herbs, seeds, essential oils, and supplies geared toward the self-reliant herbalist. All herb products indicate whether they are organic, wild-crafted, or commercially grown.

Pacific Botanicals
541-479-7777
www.pacificbotanicals.com
Certified organic fresh and dried herbs sold by the pound.

Sage Woman Herbs
888-350-3911
www.sagewomanherbs.com
I like the way they indicate on each listing for bulk herbs and tinctures whether it is organic, wild-crafted, and (for tinctures) made with fresh plants. Also sells bath salts, capsules, formulas, and extracts.

EDUCATION AND ASSOCIATIONS
It would literally take a book to list all the herb classes and seminars held throughout the United States. Fortunately, the American Herbalist Guild (AHG) and the American Herb Association (AHA) have already compiled a comprehensive directory.

American Association of Naturopathic Physicians
202-237-8150
www.naturopathic.org
Provides referrals to a national network of accredited for licensed practitioners. Brochures and pamphlets.

American Botanical Council
512-926-4900
www.herbalgram.org
Nonprofit research and education organization. Publishes Herbalgram and distributes many hard-to-find botany and herbal books.

The American Herb Association
530-265-9552
www.ahaherb.com
Directories of herbal education and herb products. Quarterly newsletter.

The American Herbalist Guild
203-272-6731
www.americanherbalistsguild.com
Emphasizes and promotes the practice of herbal medicine in North America. Quarterly publication.

American Association for Health Freedom
800-230-2762
www.healthfreedom.net
Advocacy group promoting alternative health care on a grassroots and professional level.

Bio-Dynamic Farming and Gardening Association
888-516-7797
www.biodynamics.com
Advances the practice and principles of biodynamic agriculture through publications, advisory services, programs, seminars, and conferences.

Citizens for Health
612-879-7585
www.citizens.org
Grassroots information on political and market trends in alternative medicine.

Herb Growing and Marketing Network
717-393-3295
www.herbworld.com
Trade association and excellent information resource for herb businesses and serious hobbyists. Publishes an annual industry wide resource guide and a quarterly trade journal.

Herb Research Foundation
303-449-2265
www.herbs.org
Custom research services and sells information packets on over 200 common herbs. Several publications.

Kerr Center for Sustainable Agriculture
918-647-9123
www.kerrcenter.com
A non-profit organization that provides support, research, and education on sustainable agriculture.

Lady Bird Johnson Wildflower Center
512-292-4100
www.wildflower.org
Dedicated to the preservation and reestablishment of native flora. Provides information on propagation, seed collection, wildlife gardening, and planting in your geographic area.

The Northeast Herbal Association
www.northeastherbal.org
Publishes one of my favorite newsletters (it reads as an ongoing discussion among herbalists) and works to educate and promote herbalism throughout the eastern United States.

United Plant Savers
802-476-6467
http://unitedplantsavers.org
Devoted to replanting endangered and threatened species in the environment for non-harvestable purposes.

PERIODICALS

Acres USA: A Voice for Eco-Agriculture
800-355-5313
www.acresusa/magazines/magazine.htm
Monthly magazine. Many articles on herbs and health in an agricultural context. Excellent reading.

The Herb Companion
800-456-5835
www.herbcompanion.com
Bimonthly, full-color magazine. Also publishes Herbs for Health, which provides information about medicinal herbs.

Herbalgram: The Journal of the American Botanical Council
512-926-4900
www.herbalgram.org

The Wild Food Forum
www.edibleplants.com/wff/wffhome.htm
Excellent newsletter about edible and medicinally useful plants.

INDEX

Page references in *italics* indicate illustrations.

Cradle cap, 133
Cramps, 41, 120–21
Cuts and scrapes, 41, 42, 64, 113–14
Cycle of life, *104*

D

Dandelion *(Taraxacum officinale)*,
34–35, *34*
Decongestants, 43, 63, 64
Dehydration, 56, 121–22
Dental ailments, 137–38
Depression, 36, 40–41, 57, 140
Detoxification, 34, 121
Diaper rash, 64, 133
Diarrhea, 33, 39, 41, 56, 121–22
Diet and chronic illnesses, 103–4
Digestive bitters, 55
Digestive disorders, 32, 34–35, 36,
38, 74
Disinfectants, 93
Diuretics, 34–35
Drying herbs, 12–13, *13*
Dysentery, 32, 56

E

Earaches, 37, 122–23
Eczema, 37, 42, 65, 134
Equipment, *23*
    jars, 23–24
    labels, 23
    mortars and pestles, 24–25, *25*
    notebooks, 22–23
    presses, 24, *24*
    saucepans, 25
    scales, 25, *25*
    strainers, 24
Essiac, 153–54
Evening primrose oil, 65
Eye strain/irritation, 125

F

Fatigue, 33, 38, 72, 141
Fevers, 33, 34, 35, 36, 125–26
Field guides, 8
First aid, 97
Flu, 33, 35, 55, 126–27
Food poisoning, 33
Foot pain, 63
Freezing herbs, 13

Frostbite, 127
Fungal infections, 41, 42, 57, 144–45

G

Garlic *(Allium sativum)*, 35, *35*
Gathering plants. *See* Plant gathering
Ginger *(Zingiber officinale)*, 35, *35*
Glycerin, 20–21
Gray hair, 127–28

H

Hangovers, 35, 65, 121
Hay fever, 107–9
Headaches, 36, 37, 38, 128–29
Heartburn, 34, 36, 131–32
Heart problems, 35, 129–30
Hemorrhoids, 130
Herbal blends, 99–100, 105–6
    for acute illnesses, 100–102
    for chronic illnesses, 103–5
Herbalism
    achieving balance, 150–51
    connecting with plants, 148–49,
    148–49
    in the information age, 155
    Native American, 151–54
    subconscious voice and, 147–48
Herbal therapy, 1–2, 43–44, 107
Herb quality
    in capsules, 17
    color and smell, 16
    in imported herbs, 16
    organic certification, 15–16
    pesticides and, 16
Herpes sores, 36
High blood pressure, 35
Honey, 21, 96

I

Illnesses. *See* Ailments/Conditions
Impetigo, 57
Indigestion, 37, 41, 55, 74, 131–32
Infections, 133
    bladder, 134–35
    fungal, 41, 42, 57, 144–45
    umbilical, 133
Inflammations, 32, 33–34, 35, 39,
64, 133
Influenza. *See* Flu

Other Storey Titles You Will Enjoy

Herbal Antibiotics, by Stephen Harrod Buhner.
Focused, specific information on how to
use antibiotics provided by Mother Nature.
144 pages. Paper. ISBN 978-1-58017-148-9.

**The Herbal Home Spa: Naturally Refreshing Wraps, Rubs,
Lotions, Masks, Oils, and Scrubs,** by Greta Breedlove.
A collection of easy-to-create personal care products that
rival potions found at exclusive spas and specialty shops.
208 pages. Paper. ISBN 978-1-58017-005-5.

Herbal Remedy Gardens, by Dorie Byers.
More than 35 illustrated plans for easy-to-maintain
container and backyard herbal gardens.
224 pages. Paper. ISBN 978-1-58017-095-6.

Herbal Tea Gardens, by Marietta Marshall Marcin.
A tea lover's gardening bible, complete growing
instructions and recipes for blending and brewing.
192 pages. Paper. ISBN 978-1-58017-106-9.

Organic Body Care Recipes, by Stephanie Tourles.
Homemade, herbal formulas for glowing skin, hair,
and nails, plus a vibrant self.
384 pages. Paper. ISBN 978-1-58017-676-7.

Perfumes, Splashes & Colognes, by Nancy M. Booth.
Step-by-step, illustrated instructions for making personal
blends with herbs, essential oils, and fragrance oils.
176 pages. Paper. ISBN 978-0-88266-985-4.

Rosemary Gladstar's Herbal Recipes for Vibrant Health.
A practical compendium of herbal lore and know-how
for wellness, longevity, and boundless energy.
408 pages. Paper. ISBN 978-1-60342-078-5.

These and other books from Storey Publishing are available
wherever quality books are sold or by calling 1-800-441-5700.
Visit us at *www.storey.com.*